Endothelial Cell Vesicles

Progress in Applied Microcirculation
Mikrozirkulation in Forschung und Klinik

Vol. 9

Series Editors
K. Messmer, Heidelberg; *F. Hammersen*, Munich

KARGER

Basel · München · Paris · London · New York · New Delhi · Singapore · Tokyo · Sydney

Proceedings of a Workshop at the Third World Congress for Microcirculation,
Oxford/United Kingdom, September 9–14, 1984

Endothelial Cell Vesicles

Volume Editors
F. Hammersen, Munich; *D. H. Lewis,* Linköping

46 figures and 20 tables, 1985

KARGER

Basel · München · Paris · London · New York · New Delhi · Singapore · Tokyo · Sydney

Progress in Applied Microcirculation
Mikrozirkulation in Forschung und Klinik

National Library of Medicine, Cataloging in Publication

Endothelial cell vesicles: proceedings of a workshop at the Third World Congress for Microcirculation, Oxford/United Kingdom, September 9–14, 1984 / volume editors, F. Hammersen, D. H. Lewis. – Basel; New York: Karger, 1985. – (Progress in applied microcirculation = Mikrozirkulation in Forschung und Klinik; vol. 9)
Includes index.
1. Biological Transport – congresses
2. Capillary – permeability – congresses
3. Endothelium – cytology – congresses I. Hammersen, Frithjof II. Lewis, David H. III. World Congress for Microcirculation (3rd: 1984 Oxford, Oxfordshire) IV. Series: Progress in applied microcirculation; vol. 9
ISBN 3-8055-4070-1
WI PR666FI v.9
QS 532.5.E7 E565 1984

Printed in Germany by Mühlberger GmbH, D-8900 Augsburg
ISBN 3-8055-4070-1

Contents

Preface

With the very beginning of the enormous impact of electron microscopy on cell biology, vesicles of ca. 500–700 Å in outer diameter were recognized as a regular component of a variety of endothelial cells. In his famous and frequently, yet in most cases erroneously cited short report on these structures (the correct title of the journal is: J. appl. Physics and not J. appl. Physiol.), Dr. *Palade* assumed even at that time (1953) that the vesicles 'may represent a system for transporting fluids across the capillary wall and may account for the high permeability rate of the capillaries' by means of a vesicular shuttle. This suggestion established the 'ferry boat theory' of vesicular transport. At the beginning, most physiologists rejected this new kind of a transport mechanism on the grounds of quantitative considerations, until electron dense tracers with a wide spectrum of molecular weights became increasingly available which definitely established 'vesicular transport' as a biologically significant means for the normal transendothelial movement of plasma proteins. In addition, the vesicles appeared to be the most likely candidate for the so-called large pores introduced by *Pappenheimer* into the permeability discussion. Although several laboratories published experimental evidence indicating that a vesicular shuttle cannot be the correlate of the 'large pores', the majority favored 'vesicular transport' as a realistic mechanism to explain the normally occurring transcapillary transport of high molecular substances, particularly of plasma proteins.

This long held assumption became substantially questioned, because the analysis of ultrathin serial sections resulted in a new three-dimensional model of vesicular organization. According to this all vesicles are gathered into small intercommunicating clusters of racemose configuration which either open to the luminal or to the abluminal surface, but never simultaneously to both. So called 'free' vesicles are absent.

The immediate opposite of this is a hypothesis named 'transcytosis'. This designates an active, continuous process of vesicle fusion by which either transendothelial channels or fenestrae are formed. Since the majority of both structures is equipped with size-limiting structures, such as delicate diaphragms and localized strictures, fenestrae and channels are assumed to be the structural correlates of the 'small pores', whereas the few truly 'open' channels and fenestrae (without diaphragms) represent the 'large pores'.

To evaluate the present state of the art, we have gathered experts from different laboratories from all over the world who employ different experimental models and techniques to achieve a better understanding of the structure-function interrelationship of capillary endothelial cell vesicles.

Munich/Linköping,
September 1985

F. Hammersen
D. H. Lewis

List of Contributors and Invited Discussants

J. F. Bernaudin
Université Paris
Val de Marne
Faculté de Médecine de Créteil
Département d'Enseignement et
de Recherche d'Histologie et Embryologie
8, rue de Général Sarrail
F-94010 Créteil Cedex (France)

J. R. Casley-Smith
Microcirculation Research Unit
University of Adelaide
Box 498 G. P. O.
Adelaide
South Australia 5001 (Australia)

G. Clough
Department of Physiology
and Biophysics
St. Mary's Hospital
Medical School
London (England)

D. O. DeFouw
Department of Anatomy
UMDNJ-New-Jersey Medical School
100 Bergen Street
Newark, NJ 07103 (USA)

J. Frøkjær-Jensen
Laboratory of Neurobiology
The Marine Biological Laboratory
Woods Hole, MA 02543 (USA)

F. Hammersen
Department of Anatomy
Technical University Munich
Biedersteiner Str. 29
D-8000 Munich (FRG)

D. H. Lewis
Linköping University
Clinical Research Center
S-581 85 Linköping (Sweden)

C. C. C. O'Morchoe
Department of Anatomy and Pathology
University of Illinois
College of Medicine
at Urbana-Champaign
190 Medical Sciences Buildings
506 South Mathews
Urbana, IL 61801 (USA)

G. G. Pietra
Anatomic Pathology Division
Hospital of the University
of Pennsylvania
34th and Spruce Streets
Philadelphia, PA 19104 (USA)

U. S. Ryan
Department of Medicine D-58
University of Miami
School of Medicine
P. O. Box 016960
Miami, FL 33101 (USA)

E. E. Schneeberger
Department of Pathology
Massachusetts General Hospital
Harvard Medical School
Boston, MA 02114 (USA)

St. M. Shea
Department of Pathology
UMDNJ-Rutgers Medical School
Piscataway, NJ 08854 (USA)

A. E. Taylor
Department of Physiology
College of Medicine
University of South Alabama
Mobile, AL 36688 (USA)

R. C. Tripathi
Eye Research Laboratories
The University of Chicago
939 East 57th Street
Chicago, IL 60637 (USA)

R. C. Wagner
School of Life and Health Sciences
University of Delaware
Newark, DE 19716 (USA)

S. K. Williams
Department of Physiology
Jefferson Medical College
Thomas-Jefferson-University
Philadelphia, PA 19140 (USA)

Prog. appl. Microcirc., vol. 9, pp. 1–5 (Karger, Basel 1985)

Application of High Voltage Electron Microscopy (HVEM) to Visualize the Three-Dimensional Structure of the Vesicular System in Thick Sections

R. C. Wagner

School of Life and Health Sciences, University of Delaware, Newark, Del., USA

Introduction

Endothelial vesicles are conspicuous and compelling features of the walls of continuous capillaries. Intravital tracer methods indicate that they mediate bidirectional transport of large solutes across capillary walls [1, 4]. The mechanism by which it is accomplished, however, remains elusive since it is difficult to extrapolate their dynamic activity from static ultrastructural images. Caveolae and compound vesicular profiles suggest fission and fusion events caught in stopped-time. Conventional electron microscopy of thin sections is limited to two-dimensional profiles, however, and the relationships of vesicles outside of the plane of section is not perceived.

Three-dimensional information on the vesicular system has been provided by reconstruction of serial sections [2, 3] and tannic acid mordanting of compartments open to the cell surface [6]. These methods have revealed that many vesicular profiles which would otherwise be construed as discrete cytoplasmic entities actually communicate via intervesicular fusions with the extracellular compartment. The extent of this error in interpretation and its meaning regarding vesicular function has prompted much current debate. The efficacy of aldehyde fixatives in preserving the vesicular system in its natural configuration has also been questioned [5].

An alternative method of procuring three-dimensional information about the capillary wall is by stereoscopic viewing of high voltage electron micrographs of thick sections. This approach obviates some of the rigors and sampling limitations of serial section reconstruction by permitting visualization of vesicle associations in a single image. Under proper conditions, three-dimensional images of complex structures several vesicle diameters thick can be viewed in their entirety.

Material and Methods

Albino rats were perfused with glutaraldehyde (1%) and formaldehyde (1%) in 0.1 M tyrodes cacodylate buffer (pH 7.1) for 15 min followed by tannic acid and glutaraldehyde (1% each) for 15 min. The diaphragm muscle was then removed, cut into strips parallel to the muscle fibers, and immersed in tannic acid and glutaraldehyde for 30 min to allow penetration of the tannic acid into the interstitial spaces. The tissue was then postfixed in 1% OsO_4, dehydrated, and embedded in Spurr's medium. Thick 0.5–1.0 μm sections (green interference color) were cut on glass knives, placed on folding grids (150 mesh) and counterstained with uranyl acetate (1 h at 50 °C) and lead citrate (1 h at room temperature). The sections were examined with the 1.3 MEV electron microscope at the HVEM facility of the New York State Department of Health, Albany, New York. Stereopair micrographs were taken between 12 K and 100 K magnification and at tilt angle differentials of between 4 and 8 degrees.

Results

Stereoimages of thick sections through diaphragm muscle capillary walls exhibit a remarkable amount of depth and allow perception of relationships between vesicular structures in their entirety (figs. 1 and 2). Tannic acid mordanting is particularly evident in association with residual serum protein, RBCs, attached caveolae, and the basement membrane. The basement membrane appears as a soft, translucent feltwork through which underlying caveolae can be seen. The contrast differential between tannic acid-labeled and unlabeled compartments is not as pronounced as in thin sections. This is probably due to the fact that an enhanced amount of intrinsic contrast is imparted by overlapping structures and that membranous structures are viewed throughout their depth.

Three-dimensional perception of stereopairs involves the neurological phenomenon of cortical fusion and thus cannot be conveyed directly in two-dimensional space. Graphic interpretations can be made, however, which facilitates presentation of data (fig. 3). Such analysis reveals that a variety of simple and compound vesicular forms are present but not all are

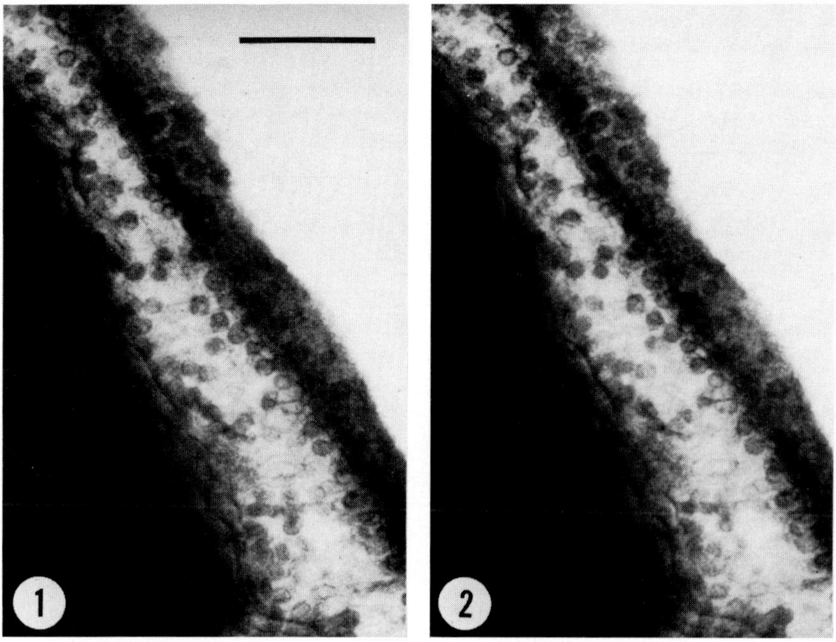

Figs. 1 and 2. High voltage stereopair micrographs of a thick section through the wall of a diaphragm muscle capillary. The basement membrane appears as a fine feltwork through which underlying caveolae can be seen. The coexistence of free and attached vesicular structures is clearly evident. 37,000×. Bar represents 0.5 μm.

conjoined or maintain connections with the cell surface. Discrete and internalized vesicular structures are readily detectable although at apparently lower incidence than would be assumed from thin sections.

Discussion

The usefulness of stereomicroscopy for three-dimensional analysis of the vesicular system depends upon the section thickness and the relative density of vesicles within the section. Thin sections less than one vesicle diameter thick (fig. 4 a) permit visualization of vesicle association only in one plane. If the section is too thick or the vesicle density too high (fig. 4 c), overlapping of vesicular structures obscures their interrelationships and any connections between vesicular compartments remain hidden.

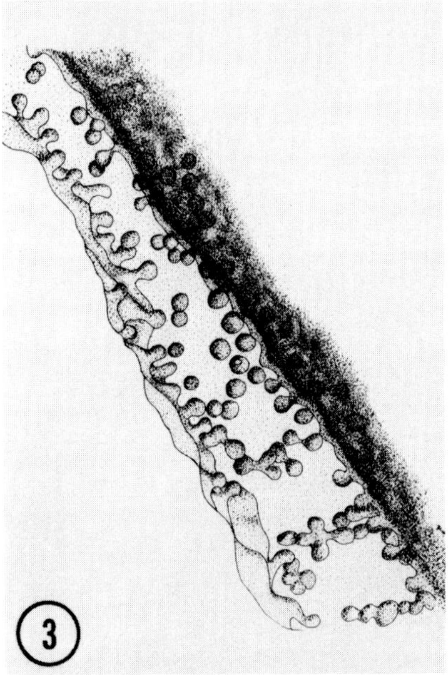

3

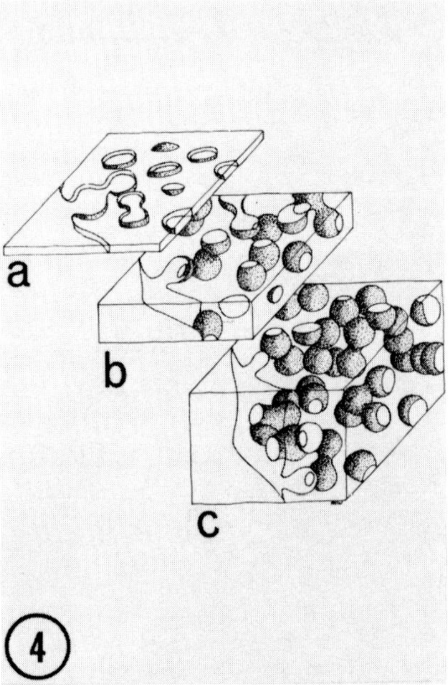

4

Fig. 3. An interpretive illustration of the three-dimensional image generated by the stereopair of figures 1 and 2. In areas where interrelationships are not obscured by overlapping structures, vesicle forms can be seen in their entirety. Internalized single vesicles are present as well as portions of spheres transected by the plane of section.

Fig. 4. An illustration of sections of three different thicknesses demonstrating the importance of both section thickness and vesicle density in the ability to perceive interrelationships. Thin sections (*a*) reveal associations in only one plane. In sections which are too thick or contain too many vesicles per unit volume (*c*), relationships are obscured by overlapping structures. The proper relation between thickness and vesicle density (*b*) is most ideal for perceiving the three-dimensional structure of the vesicular system.

Thus, it is not always possible to classify vesicles as simple, compound, free, or attached, which precludes meaningful morphometric analysis. However, under ideal conditions of section thickness and vesicle density (fig. 4 b), many vesicle forms and their associations can be viewed in their entirety.

Although no definite information about vesicle dynamics can be deduced from static EM images, a constant state of flux between vesicular compartments should result in some discrete vesicular entities in fixed tissue. These are readily detectable in thick sections through the walls of diaphragm capillaries. The shapes and varieties of vesicular forms present suggest membrane compartments in transition. Repeated segregation and reconnection of vesicular compartments with each other and the capillary surface may provide a discontinuous pathway for large solutes across the capillary wall.

Summary

High voltage electron microscopy (HVEM) of thick sections of diaphragm muscle capillaries was employed to visualize the three-dimensional structure of the vesicular system. Stereological viewing of micrographs taken at different angles of stage tilt provided for direct visualization of entire vesicular structures. A variety of simple and compound vesicles are present but not all are conjoined or maintain connections with the cell surface. Completely internalized vesicles are present although at a lower incidence than might be assumed from thin sections.

Acknowledgment

Supported by PHS Grant HL 16666 to RCW and PHS Grant RRO 129 to the New York State High Voltage Electron Microscopy Facility as a National Biotechnology Resource.

References

1 Bruns, R.; Palade, G.: Studies on blood capillaries. II. Transport of ferritin molecules across the wall of muscle capillaries. J. Cell Biol. *37:* 277–299 (1968).

2 Bundgaard, M.; Hagman, P.; Crone, C.: The three-dimensional organization of plasmalemmal vesicular profiles in the endothelium of heart capillaries. Microvasc. Res. *25:* 358–368 (1983).

3 Frøkjær-Jensen, J.: Three-dimensional organization of plasmalemmal vesicles in endothelial cells. An analysis by serial sectioning of frog mesenteric capillaries. J. Ultrastruct. Res. *73:* 9–20 (1980).

4 Johansson, B.: Permeability of muscle capillaries to interstitially injected ferritin. Microvasc. Res. *16:* 362–368 (1978).

5 McGuire, P.; Twietmeyer, J.: Morphology of rapidly frozen aortic endothelial cells: Glutaraldehyde fixation increases the number of caveolae. Circulation Res. *53:* 424–429 (1983).

6 Wagner, R.; Robinson, C.: Tannic acid tracer analysis of permeability pathways in the rete mirabile: Demonstration of the discreteness of endothelial vesicles. J. Ultrastruct. Res. *81:* 37–46 (1982).

R. C. Wagner, PhD, School of Life and Health Sciences, University of Delaware, Newark, DE 19716 (USA)

Prog. appl. Microcirc., vol. 9, pp. 6–20 (Karger, Basel 1985)

Vesicular Form and Fusion – As Revealed by Freeze-Immobilization and Stereoscopy of Semi-thin Sections:

Implications for Permeation via these Structures

J. R. Casley-Smith

Microcirculation Research Unit, University of Adelaide, Adelaide, Australia

Introduction

The small, smooth vesicles of blood vascular and lymphatic endothelium are very obvious structures. Their morphology and its implications for permeability have caused great controversy [reviewed: 3, 11, 17, 19, 25, 31, 35]. In general the controversy revolves around two main considerations:

(1) Are there many vesicles lying free in the cytoplasm, or do they almost all join together, opening at one side of the cell or the other?

(2) Are there many thoroughfare channels, i.e., channels formed by one, or a chain of vesicles, opening on the two surfaces of the endothelium?

It is generally agreed that, if many free vesicles do exist and if many thoroughfare channels do not, the vesicles slowly ferry macromolecules across the endothelial barrier, acting as the large pores in continuous (but not in fenestrated) capillaries [reviewed: 11, 25, 31]. It is also generally agreed that they would be randomly propelled by their Brownian motion, without the need for cellular energy [11, 15, 18, 31]. This has actually been observed, in vivo, with small complex-vesicles [6]. This thermodynamic motion also accounts [11] for vesicles fused with a plasma membrane separating from it (or other vesicles) and free ones joining such membranes.

If, however, there are only a very few free vesicles this transport would be unlikely to occur in sufficient amounts. Again, if there were many thoroughfare channels, these could account for the large pores – without the need for the vesicular hypothesis. The numbers found by the *Simionescu*'s [28, 29] – about 1 per 4 capillary cross-sections – are sufficient even to account for the small pores [*Casley-Smith,* 1977, unpub.]. These possibilities will be examined.

Results and Discussion

Are Many Vesicles Free?

Tannic acid has been used to label all vesicles continuous with the cell surfaces. It shows that about 50% of the apparently free ones are continuous with the exterior [19, 26, 30–35]. The remainder, however, are actually free – especially in thicker endothelium.

By contrast, some workers [3–5, 16, 17] consider that tannic acid labels all (or very nearly all) vesicles, and that these form static, complex, racemose structures – opening at one (but not both) surfaces of the endothelium. This conclusion has been attacked [31, 34] on the grounds that if tannic acid penetrates endothelial cells, via breaks in their walls, all vesicles will be labelled. This labelling will not occur just on the interior of the vesicle, (as in the case of those which are labelled when the plasma membranes are intact), but on both lamellae of their unit-membranes [26, 30, 33]. Such spurious labelling has been reported [34] for the illustrations which seem to demonstrate that all vesicles are labelled. This implies that the cells are damaged during processing – perhaps by the long fixation periods used (see below).

Some other workers also found considerable amounts of labelling with tracers after exposing the cells to them well after fixation might be expected to have finished [20, reviewed: 3, 17, 31]. However, it will be pointed out later that fixation actually takes a long time. In addition, many of the labelled vesicles must have filled in a retrograde manner, from the interstitial tissue; this is because so many were ablumenal vesicles. Hence, this evidence is dubious!

Another argument has been advanced in favour of vesicles being static objects [12, 17]: those adjacent to the lumen are often filled with plasma; those adjacent to the ablumenal surface are not. However, if vesicular motion is random, one must expect most of those which leave one surface will return to it – not to the opposite one [11, 15, 18]. Hence, this argument is also invalid.

Conventional thin sections (50–60 nm) show that many of the vesicles are apparently free. Serial sectioning, using these, showed many free vesicles [24]. However, serial reconstructions from very thin (15 nm) sections suggest that this appearence is an artefact, and that almost all vesicles actually unite with others – eventually opening at one or the other surface of the cell [3–5, 16, 17]. This conclusion has been criticized because ultra-thin sections allow only a very small volume of tissue to be examined, with the possibilities of sampling errors [34]; on the other hand, many thousands of vesicles have been examined in this way in some 8 μm^3 of endothelium [3], so one must doubt the validity of this particular criticism. Nevertheless, other evidencc (apart from that mentioned above) does indicate that many free vesicles do, in fact, exist.

Stereoscopy of semi-thin (0.5–1 μm) sections has been performed with high-voltage transmission electron microscopy [34]. This permits many more vesicles to be studied than is possible with the very laborious method of ultra-thin serial sectioning. Many vesicles were found to be completely free.

Why are so many free ones found with this method, but not with serial ultra-thin sections? Apart from the volumes of tissue involved (above), one possibility is that only a portion of the ultra-thin sections is actually observed. Lead only stains 4 nm into the section [14]. Hence, only about 25 % of the thickness of even ultra-thin sections is actually observed. They really represent, not a block of tissue, but only slices of it – separated by 3-times their widths. On the other hand, published series [4, 5, 16, 17] make it seem unlikely that many discontinuous vesicles would be mistaken for continuous ones.

One possibly very important methodological difference is that those workers who find no free vesicles [3–5, 16, 17] fix, with glutaraldehyde, for much longer times than those [19, 21, 24, 25, 30–34] who find many free ones after tannic acid labelling, etc. The former fix for 15–20 h; the latter fix for 15–60 min. Could this cause the difference? Perhaps the long fixations promote the fusion of adjacent membranes and then cause holes to form – both as a result of excessive cross-linking and contraction of the proteins in and around the membranes? These would explain both the spurious tannic acid labelling and the lack of free vesicles in serial ultra-thin sections. Other artefacts of chemical fixation are discussed later.

Do Thoroughfare Channels Exist?

Simionescu et al. [28, 29] found what appeared to be many transendothelial, thoroughfare channels – right through the endothelium of the capillaries of rat and mouse diaphragms. These consisted of a vesicle opening at both sides of the cell, or a chain of several, fused vesicles doing this. Heme-peptides and horseradish peroxidase were clearly continuous: inside the lumen, through the channels, and outside the vessels. The possibility that overlapping vesicles might appear artefactually joined was largely excluded by tilting techniques – although three-dimensional geometry shows that the tilting employed would not have been sufficient in all cases [15]. Also, some single vesicles joined both plasma membranes, with continuity between all three membranes.

This had indeed been hypothesized by *Bruns and Palade* [1]. From time to time, all workers who have looked at many vesicles have seen appearances suggesting such channels [reviewed: 28, 29, 31, 35]. They are usually dismissed as too few to be of any importance, but the numbers found by *Simionescu* et al. [28, 29] are far too many to be considered trivial (see above), although one may assume that diaphragms cause molecular sieving. Some workers have also found such channels, but most, who have searched for them very carefully, did not find them – or found them only very rarely [reviewed: 3, 11, 17, 31]. These observations (for both points of view) were made using chemical fixation.

Problems of Chemical Fixation

Apart from artefacts caused by very long fixation (above), chemical fixation (or, rather, immobilization) may cause others. It is a very slow process – taking nearly a minute – to prevent visible Brownian motion and saltatory movements, even when applied directly onto tissue culture cells [2]. There is evidence that fixation is not complete until 1–2 hours have passed [reviewed: 11]. These times may be compared with the suggestion, for which there is considerable evidence [11, 12, 15, 18, 21, 31], that vesicles can detach, traverse the cell and fuse with the plasma membrane again – all in a matter of a few seconds. So, chemical fixation could cause very serious artefacts indeed.

A fused vesicle – which would normally detach many times during the chemical immobilization period – is likely to be retained, during this process, still fused to the plasma membrane by cross-linking by the fixative. Yet its anti-membranous surface would still be able to fuse with the opposite plasma membrane, or another vesicle. (The vesicle, the membranes, and indeed all the cellular contents would still be subject to considerable Brownian movements until much time had passed, and so could easily contact each other). Such fusion would be encouraged by the fixation process. Thus, thoroughfare channels could be formed, as would additional complex, racemose vesicles. The formation of both would be increased if any agglutinable material were contained in them, *viz.* plasma proteins or the tracers so often added during these experiments.

Freeze-Immobilization

An alternative method of immobilization of the tissue is to use freezing (often associated with fixation, during substitution of the ice by acetone). The fixation actually occurs over many hours, but the structures are meanwhile immobilized by the ice. The wave of freezing actually crosses an endothelial cell in some 0.02 s [10].

Using this technique [10], no thoroughfare channels were found (table I). This was in spite of using the identical tissue (mouse diaphragm) in which they were so frequently reported after chemical fixation [29].

On the other hand, in lung capillaries *Mazzone and Kornblau* [22] found 11 thoroughfare channels in freeze-immobilized tissue, compared with 18 in chemically-fixed (both per 80 micrographs – apparently of complete capillary cross-sections). (This difference is not significant). While these authors concluded that such channels were 'not abundant' in this site, in fact this is a very similar proportion to that found by *Simionescu* et al. [28, 29] – and could account for both the large and the small pore systems (see above)! Unfortunately, they gave no details of the criteria they used to identify a thoroughfare channel, nor to exclude artefacts (by tilting, etc.); such methods are essential, except for single vesicles opening to both sides, otherwise overlapping vesicles may appear to communicate when they do not. Also, they used rather low magnifications (38,000 ×). From these facts, and because of the absence of such channels, even in the site where they were very common with chemical fixation (above), it seems best to regard this report with caution.

An additional problem of chemical fixation is that the shapes of vesicles could easily be distorted. *Palade and Bruns* [24] considered that fus-

Table I[a]. Mouse diaphragm blood capillaries. Results for freezing, compared with chemical immobilization – Thin sections

	Freeze immobilization	Chemical immobilization[b]	
		This site [8]	Reported range
Vesicles – free[e]			
RMS internal diam (nm)	54.9 (2.51) *500*	52.5 (1.40) *300*[NS]	50–65
Nos./μm² of lumenal surface[c,e]	70.3 (9.51) *100*	155 (37.6) *20**	50–155
Nos./μm³ of cytoplasm[c,e]	395 (90.6) *100*	700 (78.8) *40***	350–700
Vesicles – attached			
Internal diam. of necks (nm)	37.2 (1.80) *500*	14–17 (0.89) *300****	14–17
Depth (nm)	48.2 (2.86) *500*	87.7 (1.90) *300****	80–90
No./μm² of plasma membrane[c,e]	53.8 (3.17) *200*	136 (11.2) *60****	60–140
No./μm³ of cytoplasm[c,e]	302 (58.8) *200*	531 (44.2) *40***	300–600
Proportion with diaphragms	0.20 (0.019) *500*		
Proportion with partial diaphs.	0.26 (0.020) *500*		< 0.015***
Proportion with narrow necks	0.18 (0.017) *500*		> 0.985***
Vesicles – total[e]			
Numbers/μm² of lumenal surface	178 (6.46) *100*	427 (28.5) *20****	100–400
Numbers/μm³ of cytoplasm[d]	999 (73.0) *100*	1760 (85.8) *20****	500–1700
Thoroughfare channels per cap. cross-section	0	0	0.254[f]***

[a] Results given as means, S.E.'s (in brackets) and numbers (italics); '*' etc. have their usual statistical significance – comparing freezing and chemical fixation; [b] from references [1, 8, 11, 15, 24, 27–29, 32]; [c] x 2/pi of the measured circum. or diam. [15] to allow for random angles of sectioning and of orientation of the elliptical capillaries; [d] adjusted for random angle of sectioning and resolution [14]; [e] in peripheral zones – 0.872 (0.053) *40* of whole circumference [15]; [f] many authors record none (see text); others [28, 29] record at least 0.254.

ing vesicles were squat and wide-mouthed, while ones about to detach were tear-drop shaped. They, and others, observed many more of the latter (table II). If chemical fixation causes delayed fission, many of the former would remain to take the latter shape – but would not detach. Freezing immobilization greatly reduced the proportions of vesicles in the fission-mode (with narrow necks – table I), compared with those in the fusion-mode [9, 10] – using two different freeze-substitution techniques (figs. 1, 2). This alteration can also be seen in the illustrations of *Mazzone* et al. [23], although they did not comment on it.

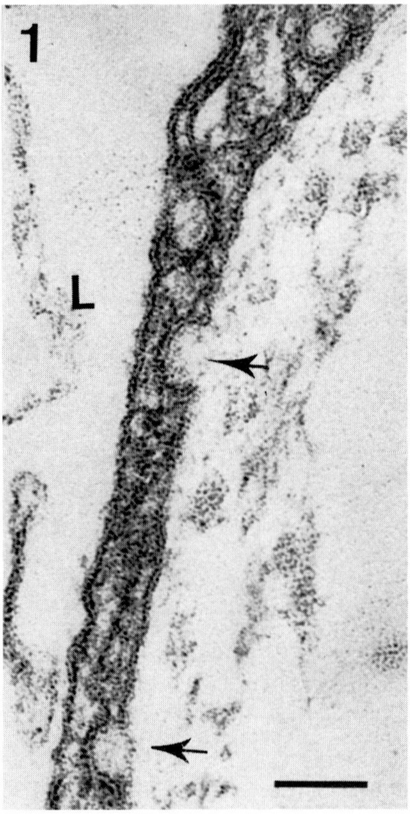

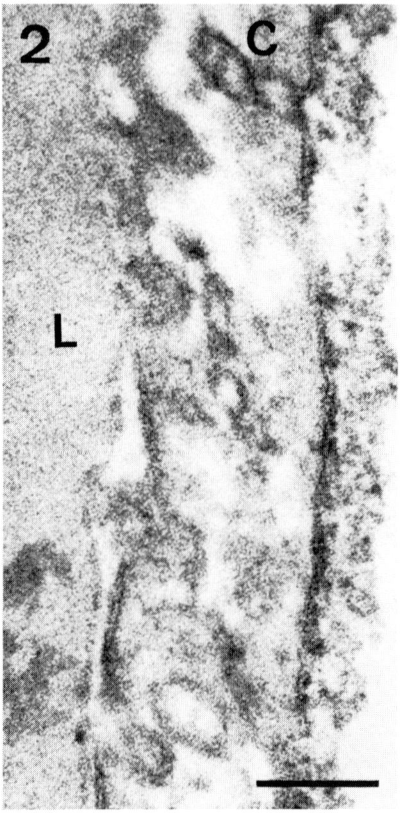

Fig. 1. Endothelium after freeze-substitution, without the injection of tracer. Three attached vesicles are shown. Two (arrows) are in the fusion-mode. Bar represents 0.1 μm; 120,000 ×; adapted from [10].

Fig. 2. As for figure 1, but 30 s after the injection of Na ferrocyanide into the blood. It is present in the lumen, outside the vessel (probably from an adjacent junction), in lumenal and ablumenal attached vesicles, and in some apparently 'free' ones. A complex vesicle (C) is present. Bar represents 0.1 μm; 160,000 ×; adapted from [10].

Almost all other workers have also observed many more attached vesicles in the fission-mode than in the fusion-mode, when using chemical fixation. The sole exception has been those working with ultra-thin serial sections [17], who consider that a single vesicle exhibits both forms – depending on how much is included in the section. This does not avoid the fact that there are very great differences in the proportions of the two forms observed in thin sections following the two methods of immobiliza-

Table II[a]. Mouse diaphragm blood capillaries. Results for stereoscopy of semi-thin sections compared with thin sections

Kind of Immobilization	Freezing	Freezing	Chemical[b]
Section Thickness:	Semi-thin (Stereoscopy)	Thin [8]	Thin
Free vesicles – per µm² lumenal surface[c]			
As single vesicles	30.5 (5.51) *25*		13–50 {*18*}
As part of complex vesicles	5.10 (2.34) *25*		4.5–10[e]
Total free vesicles	35.6 (6.00) *25*	70.3 (9.51) *100***	17–60
Uncertain if free or not	10.3 (4.23) *25*		
Free vesicles – per µm³ of cytoplasm[c]			
As single vesicles	169 (27.2) *25*		63–205 {*302*}
As part of complex vesicles	25.7 (11.1) *25*		30–150
Total free vesicles	195 (29.4) *25*	395 (90.6) *100**	93–355
Uncertain if free or not	68.7 (25.2) *25*		
Attached vesicles – per µm² lumenal surface[c]			
As single vesicles	90.1 (6.43) *25*		60–92
As part of complex vesicles	28.3 (14.4) *25*		30–63[e]
Total attached vesicles	118 (15.8) *25*	53.8 (3.17) *200****	90–155
Attached vesicles – per µm³ of cytoplasm[c]			
As single vesicles	620 (40.7) *25*		300–450
As part of complex vesicles	125 (90.0) *25*		120–250
Total attached vesicles	745 (98.8) *25*	302 (58.8) *200****	420–700
Total vesicles / µm² of surface	164 (19.0) *25*	178 (6.46) *100*[NS]	107–215
Total vesicles / µm³ cytoplasm	1009 (111) *25*	999 (73.0) *100***	513–952
Thoroughfare channels per cap. cross-section	0	0	0.254[d]

[a] Results and significances as for table I; [b] from [32] for fat capillaries, using tannic acid to label non-free vesicles; results from capillaries in rat diaphragm muscle [34] are shown in brackets {...}; [c] in peripheral zones – 0.872 (0.053) 40 of whole circumference [15]; [d] many authors record none (see text); others [28, 29] record at least 0.254; [e] calculated, assuming a mean of 3 vesicles per complex, racemose structure.

tion. Some drastic difference must be present between them; an artefact of chemical fixation is the simplest explanation.

There appear to be other alterations of the vesicles induced by chemical fixation. *Mazzone and Kornblau* [22] found many more complex, racemose vesicles after chemical fixation – supporting the concept that this promotes fusion and interferes with fission. (This finding is confirmed here, page 13 – table II).

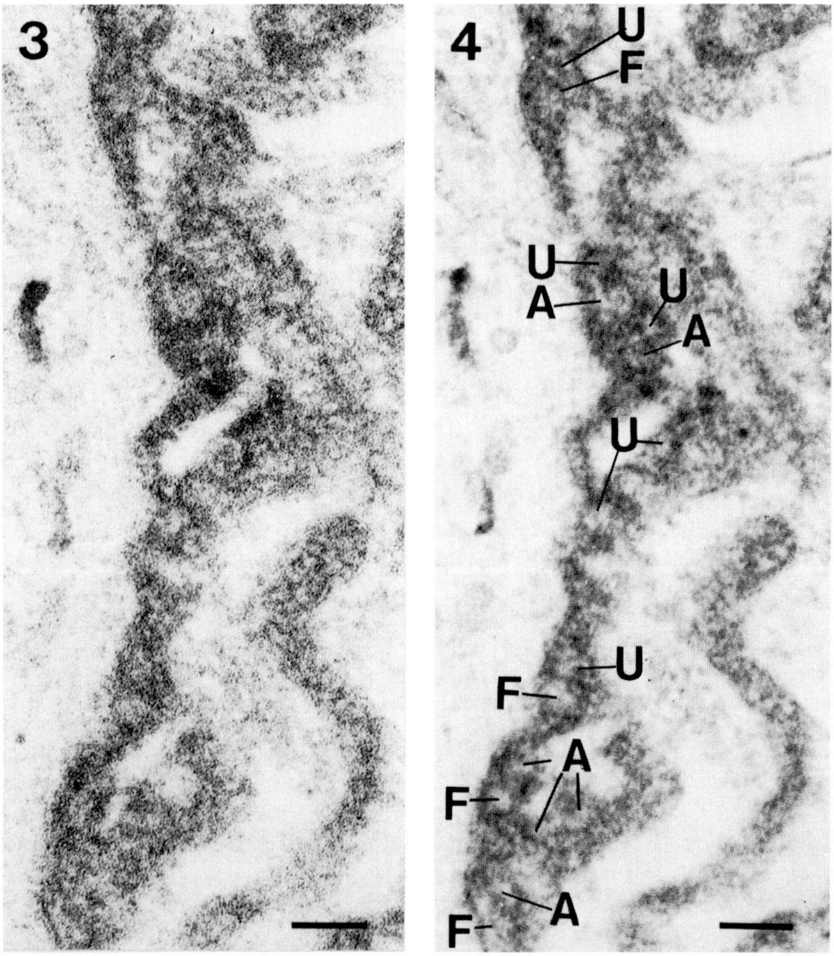

Figs. 3 and 4. A stereo-pair (stereo-angle 20°) of a 0.38 μm thick section. There are many vesicles, single and complex. Some are free (F); some are attached (A) – often via others; some are uncertain (U). Bars represent 0.1 μm each; 100,000 ×.

These workers [22] also found that vesicular volumes and numbers were both moderately increased by chemical fixation, as compared with those found after freeze-substitution. I did not notice these in my studies [9, 10]. However, now, it is evident that the numbers after chemical fixation [8] were about twice as great as after freeze-immobilization [10] – in the same species and tissue (table I). On the other hand, no significant differences in the diameters of the free vesicles were seen, between the two methods, in my studies.

It is very important to note that freeze-substitution does not reveal any other significant differences between chemically-fixed and freeze-immobilized tissue, either in blood vessels or initial lymphatics [9, 10]. In particular, the endothelial intercellular junctions [10] show the same forms, dimensions and proportions of close (narrow) regions, as compared with tight. The open junctions of the initial lymphatics, and the variations of protein concentration of the lymph, are as they appear after chemical fixation [9].

If an innocuous, ionic-sized tracer (ferro-cyanide) is introduced into the blood, this can be precipitated at the same time as the tissue is fixed – during the substitution procedure. The resulting precipitate can be seen traversing the endothelial intercellular junctions [10], just as it can in chemically-fixed tissue [7]. It can also be seen [10] in vesicles attached to the lumenal plasma membrane, apparently free in the cytoplasm, and attached to the ablumenal plasma membrane (fig. 2). The latter sometimes appear even when no other tracer can be seen in the adjacent interstitial tissue, and hence, retrograde flow is very unlikely, but no complete study of this has yet been performed. Also, the apparently free vesicles have not been examined to see if they really are free.

Stereoscopy of Freeze-Substituted Semi-thin Sections

Knowing of the successful use of stereoscopy of semi-thin sections [34], I decided to repeat this – but using the freeze-substituted material. Although a high-voltage electron microscope was not available, it is possible to view moderately thick (semi-thin) sections (0.3–0.5 μm) in a conventional instrument – provided one uses long exposures and through-focus series (since it is very hard to focus accurately). Only block stains can be used.

Hence, the mouse diaphragm muscles used in previous experiments [10] were re-examined, using this technique. The methods are set out in that publication and will not be reiterated here. Essentially, nitrogen slush was poured over the diaphragms; often this was 15–60 s after the injection of Na ferrocyanide in Ringer's solution into the blood. The substituting fluid was dehydrated acetone, in which was dissolved OsO_4 (and $FeCl_3$ for the mice injected with Na ferrocyanide). Once substitution was complete, the blocks were brought to room-temperature, block-stained with uranyl acetate, embedded in araldite and (now) sectioned at between 0.3 and 0.5 μm. The sections were examined in a JEOL 100 S and photographed stereoscopically at 30,000 ×, using a tilt-angle of 20°. The magnification was checked with a grating-replica. The stereoscopic prints were examined at a final magnification of 98,000 × (Standard Error, S.E., 2,300). The section thicknesses were measured using the electron-flux through the tissue-free resin [13]. The mean thickness was 0.43 μm (S.E. 0.073).

The first goal of the study – the localization of the tracer containing vesicles – has not been achieved. This is because it was very difficult to be sure whether a vesicle contained tracer, or not. This was most surprising since this is easy with the normal thin sections. It was so often impossible to decide one way or the other that the attempt was abandoned, for the present. The relative contrast of the tracer is greatly reduced because of the over-lying cytoplasmic material and resin, as was also found in the other study [34].

However, a second goal of the study was possible: determining relationships of vesicles, to each other and to the plasma membranes (figs. 3 and 4). This was not possible in all cases; however, it was usually possible to be relatively sure. Hence, some quantitative evaluations were attempted:

Twenty-five capillaries were randomly selected from 10 animals. Their mean lumenal surface areas were 1.57 μm^2 (S. E. 0.46) and their mean volumes were 0.34 μm^3 (S. E. 0.065). (These were calculated from the thicknesses of the sections – measured as above – and the mean endothelial widths). Vesicles were counted as 'free' (single, or part of a complex, racemose, group of two or more vesicles), 'attached to a plasma membrane' (single, or complex), or 'uncertain' (whether they were free or attached). Results are shown in table II, compared with those for thin sections (freeze-immobilized, or tannic acid stained).

The number of free vesicles was approximately halved – compared with those labelled 'free' in thin sections from this freeze-immobilized tissue. However, a considerable number (about 50% of those in 50 nm sections) were still seen to be free. Some complex vesicular structures were also free. The numbers of these, both free and attached, were reduced compared with chemical fixation.

The total numbers of free vesicles were approximately similar in number to those found to be free by tannic acid labelling in fat and muscle capillaries [32–34]. (This remark, of course, excepts the results of others [3–5] who also used this stain, but found almost no free vesicles – criticism of their results has been given earlier). The total numbers of vesicles were almost identical, for freeze-immobilized material whether conventional thin sections were examined, or stereoscopy of semi-thin sections was used. However, about half of those which appear free in conventional material are actually continuous with the exterior, and thus have to be included with the attached vesicles. Again, no thoroughfare channels were found.

Conclusions

Free vesicles do exist in considerable numbers. Since they are only some 50% less than previous estimations, the various calculations made using this number [reviewed: 11, 12, 15, 31] would be substantially unaltered. Certainly, their numbers are sufficient for them to act as the large pores in continuous capillaries. This mechanism is made much more likely by the serious doubts raised about the existence of thoroughfare channels.

However, should the estimations of transit times [11, 12, 15, 31] be altered as a result? In principal, if the numbers are halved, the calculated transit times should be halved. However, this assumes that the same endothelial thicknesses are used; this may not be correct. Earlier, the number of complex attached vesicles was not appreciated. Since vesicles departing from – or discharging into – one of these, will have much shorter paths to traverse across the cell, the transit times would be reduced. (This was earlier suggested by *Loudon* et al. [21] to explain the gradient they found in vesicular labelling). Hence, the calculated transit times may well remain about the same.

It is evident that more quantitative morphological studies are needed – using freeze-immobilization techniques. These are also needed for the repetition of the earlier studies [12, 21] which attempted to visualize the passage of tracers across the endothelium in vesicles. Only in this way can the uncertainties associated with chemical fixation be overcome.

Summary

Evidence has been reviewed concerning the existence of many free vesicles (unattached to either plasma membrane, or to vesicles attached to these) and about the existence of many thoroughfare channels. It is concluded, that many free vesicles do exist, and that many thoroughfare channels do not. Chemical fixation (and immobilization) is very slow compared with the Brownian movements of vesicles and of the plasma membrane. It is likely that this greatly contributes to the artefactual findings of thoroughfare channels, to the conversion of free vesicles to attached ones, and to alterations in the morphology of the latter. In addition, long fixation times may injure membranes, allowing tannic acid to enter the cytoplasmic matrix and stain all vesicles (artefactually suggesting that none are free). Long fixation may also cause all free vesicles to become attached, so that serial ultra-thin sectioning artefactually shows that none are free. These conclusions are supported by the stereoscopy of semi-thin (0.3–0.5 μm) sections of freeze-immobilized capillaries from mouse diaphragm. As with most other studies, it was found that about 50% of the vesicles which appear free in thin sections really are free. No thoroughfare channels were seen. Freeze-immobilization is advocated for studies of vesicles.

References

1 Bruns, R. R.; Palade, G. E.: Studies on blood capillaries. J. Cell Biol. *37:* 244–276 (1968).

2 Buckley, I. K.: Studies in fixation for electron microscopy using cultured cells. Lab. Invest. *29:* 398–410 (1973).

3 Bundgaard, M.: A critical evaluation of the concept of vesicular transport across endothelial cells; in Lambert (ed.), The pathogenicity of cationic proteins, pp. 89–99 (Raven Press, New York 1983).

4 Bundgaard, M.; Crone, C.; Frøkjær-Jensen, J.: Extreme rarity of transendothelial channels in frog mesenteric capillary. J. Physiol., Lond. *291:* 38 P (1979).

5 Bundgaard, M.; Hagman, P.; Crone, C.: The three-dimensional organisation of plasmalemmal vesicular profiles in the endothelium of rat heart capillaries. Microvasc. Res. *25:* 358–368 (1983).

6 Casley-Smith, J. R.: The Brownian movements of pinocytic vesicles. J. roy. micr. Soc. *82:* 257–261 (1983).

7 Casley-Smith, J. R.: Electron microscopical study of ions through endothelium of lymphatic and blood capillaries. Q. Il exp. Physiol. *52:* 105–113 (1967).

8 Casley-Smith, J. R.: The dimensions and numbers of small vesicles in cells, endothelial and mesothelial and the significance of these for endothelial permeability. J. Microscopy, Oxford *90:* 251–269 (1969).

9 Casley-Smith, J. R.: Fine structure of lymphatics, and the varying lymph concentration, using freeze-substitution. Folia angiol. *28:* 272–279 (1980).

10 Casley-Smith, J. R.: Freeze-substitution observations on the endothelium, and the passage of ions. Microcirculation *1:* 79–109 (1981).

11 Casley-Smith, J. R.: The structure and functioning of the blood vessels, interstitial

tissues, and lymphatics; in Földi, Casley-Smith (eds.), Lymphangiology, pp. 27–164 (Schattauer, Stuttgart, New York 1983).

12 Casley-Smith, J. R.; Chin, J. C.: The passage of cytoplasmic vesicles across endothelial and mesothelial cells. J. Microscopy, Oxford *93:* 167–189 (1971).

13 Casley-Smith, J. R.; Crocker, K. W. J.: Estimation of section thickness, etc. by quantitative electron microscopy. J. Microscopy, Oxford *103:* 351–368 (1975).

14 Casley-Smith, J. R.; Davy, P.: The estimation of distances between parallel membranes on thick sections. J. Microscopy, Oxford *114:* 249–259 (1978).

15 Casley-Smith, J. R.; Green, H.; Harris, J.; Wadey, P.: Quantitative morphology of skeletal muscle capillaries in relation to permeability. Microvasc. Res. *10:* 43–64 (1975).

16 Frøkjær-Jensen, J.: Three-dimensional organization of plasmalemmal vesicles in endothelial cells. J. Ultrastruct. Res. *73:* 9–20 (1980).

17 Frøkjær-Jensen, J.: The plasmalemmal vesicular system in capillary endothelium; in Messmer, Hammersen (eds.), Structure and function of endothelial cells. Prog. appl. Microcirc., vol. 1, pp. 17–34 (Karger, Basel 1983).

18 Green, H. S.; Casley-Smith, J. R.: Calculations on passage of small vesicles across endothelium by Brownian motion. J. theor. Biol. *35:* 103–111 (1972).

19 Karnovsky, M. J.: The ultrastructural basis of transcapillary exchanges. J. gen. Physiol. *52:* 64–95 (1968).

20 Kobayashi, S.: Ferritin labelling in the fixed muscle capillary. Arch. histol. Jap. *32:* 81–86 (1970).

21 Loudon, M. F.; Michel, C. C.; White, I. F.: The labelling of vesicles in frog endothelial cells with ferritin. J. Physiol., Lond. *296:* 97–112 (1979).

22 Mazzone, R. W.; Kornblau, S. M.: Pinocytotic vesicles in the endothelium of rapidly frozen rabbit lung. Microvasc. Res. *21:* 193–211 (1981).

23 Mazzone, R. W.; Durand, C. M.; West, J. B.: Electron microscopic appearances of rapidly frozen lung. J. Microscopy, Oxford *117:* 269–284 (1979).

24 Palade, G. E.; Bruns, R. R.: Structural modulations of plasmalemmal vesicles. J. Cell Biol. *37:* 633–653 (1968).

25 Palade, G. E.; Simionescu, M.; Simionescu, N.: Structural aspect of the permeability of the microvascular endothelium. Acta physiol. Scand. (Suppl.) *463:* 81–91 (1979).

26 Simionescu, N.; Simionescu, M.: Galloyl glucoses of low molecular weight as mordant in electron microscopy. J. Cell Biol. *70:* 608–621 (1976).

27 Simionescu, M.; Simionescu, N.; Palade, G. E.: Morphometric data on the endothelium of blood capillaries. J. Cell Biol. *60:* 128–152 (1974).

28 Simionescu, M.; Simionescu, N.; Palade, G. E.: Permeability of muscle capillaries to small heme-peptides. J. Cell Biol. *64:* 586–607 (1975).

29 Simionescu, M.; Simionescu, N.; Palade, G. E.: Structural basis of permeability in sequential segments of the microvasculature. Microvasc. Res. *15:* 17–36 (1978).

30 Wagner, R. C.: Effect of tannic acid on electron images of capillary endothelial cell membranes. J. Ultrastruct. Res. *57:* 132–139 (1976).

31 Wagner, R. C., Casley-Smith, J. R.: Endothelial vesicles. Microvasc. Res. *21:* 267–298 (1981).

32 Wagner, R. C.; Casley-Smith, J. R.: The quantitative morphometry of capillaries isolated from fat. Microcirculation *1:* 177–197 (1981).

33 Wagner, R. C.; Robinson, C. S.: Tannic acid analysis of permeability pathways in capillaries of the rete mirabile. J. Ultrastruct. Res. *81:* 37–46 (1982).
34 Wagner, R. C.; Robinson, C. S.: The three-dimensional structure of the capillary wall. Microvasc. Res. (in press 1984).
35 Wolff, J. R.: Ultrastructure of terminal vascular bed as related to function; in Kaley, Altura (eds.), Microcirculation: *1*, pp. 95–130 (University Park Press, Baltimore 1979).

J. R. Casley-Smith, MD, Microcirculation Research Unit, University of Adelaide, Box 498 G. P. O., Adelaide, South Australia 5001 (Australia)

Prog. appl. Microcirc., vol. 9, pp. 21–42 (Karger, Basel 1985)

The Vesicle Controversy

J. Frøkjær-Jensen

Institute of Medical Physiology, Department A, The Panum Institute, University of Copenhagen, Copenhagen, Denmark

Introduction

A striking and exciting morphological feature of capillary endothelium is its high content of smooth plasmalemmal vesicular profiles. They were first described by *Palade* 30 years ago [26]. Numerous studies have since been performed on the function of these 'vesicles' in transcapillary exchange of macromolecules which appear to be too large to pass the intercellular clefts, the most agreed upon passageway for small solutes [1, 3, 9, 13, 21, 30, 46, 48]. The exact size of the largest molecules which may pass the intercellular clefts in non-inflamed capillaries is not clear. It is still unsettled whether molecules like albumin (40–70 Å diameter) or horseradish peroxidase (~ 50 Å diameter) may sneak through the junctions [1, 21, 40, 48]. Most investigators agree, however, that molecules of the size of ferritin (~ 120 Å diameter) are unlikely to diffuse through intact junctions since ferritin molecules are not normally seen within the junctions of ferritin perfused vessels. Still, ferritin molecules seem to pass the capillary wall and since ferritin can equally be seen in many of the vesicular profiles within the cytoplasm of the endothelial cells and in few 'abluminal' vesicles [5, 7, 8, 19, 24] an appealing conclusion is that ferritin is transported across the capillary wall through an involvement of the 'vesicles', as no other pathway seems to exist. The mode of their involvement if, indeed, they are involved, is still unclear.

In the following, I describe the three-dimensional organization of the plasmalemmal vesicular system in different endothelia, analyzed by ultrathin (~ 140 Å) serial sectioning, and discuss the implications of this organization on current models for vesicular involvement in transcapillary exchange of macromolecules. In the last part of the paper, I report on analyses of the organization of the plasmalemmal vesicular system in non-endothelial cells (mesothelial cells and pericytes). Finally, I report on recent studies which add evidence to the concept that the main function of the plasmalemmal vesicular system in endothelial cells, as in other cells rich in vesicular profiles, probably relates to a more general cell physiological function than transendothelial transport.

Results and Discussion

Three-dimensional Organization of the Plasmalemmal Vesicular System in Endothelial Cells – Analyzed by Ultrathin (~ 140 Å) Serial Sectioning

The most direct approach to analyze the organization of the vesicular system is ultrathin serial sectioning. It was first performed on frog mesenteric capillaries [12] and later on frog striated muscle capillaries [14, 15] and rat heart capillaries [4].

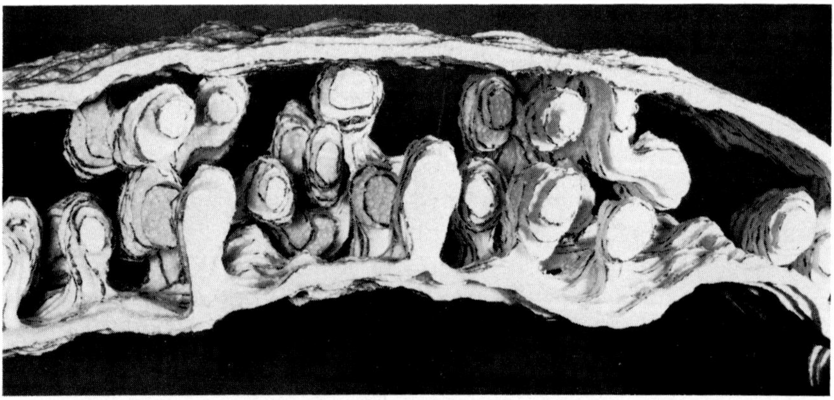

Fig. 1. Enlarged detail from a model of a segment of a frog striated muscle capillary, reconstructed from 21 ultrathin (~ 140 Å) serial sections [14]. The lumen is facing down. All vesicles belong to two separate systems of invaginations from the cell surfaces. One set connects to the luminal side, the other to the abluminal side of the capillary wall. Note how vesicles belonging to one side may be seen close to the other side of the endothelial cell. Note also the close apposition of many of the vesicles. It is unlikely that high voltage analysis of segments like this will permit full resolution of vesicle interconnections.

In all preparations, it was found that the picture of the vesicular system arising from individual conventional EM sections of capillaries is highly misleading. In individual sections, 50–70% of the total population of vesicular profiles appear without connection to the cell surface, but the ultrathin serial sectionings show that less than 1% – if any – of the apparently free smooth plasmalemmal vesicular profiles are truly free. Figure 1 illustrates the three-dimensional organization of the plasmalemmal vesicular system in a segment of an endothelial cell from a frog striated muscle capillary.

Comparison of the true distribution of single surface opening vesicles and more complex vesicular invaginations in the serial reconstructions, versus the distribution of vesicular profiles observed in individual conventional thin sections of the same capillaries, is especially important. In individual conventional thin sections of frog mesenteric and muscle capillaries, 70% of the vesicles appear without connection to the surface, 14% appear luminal and 16% appear abluminal [2, 12, 14, 15]. The ultrathin serial reconstructions, however, show that about 70% of the vesicles open directly to the luminal or abluminal surface and only about 30% communicate to the surface via a surface connected vesicle. Thus, more than

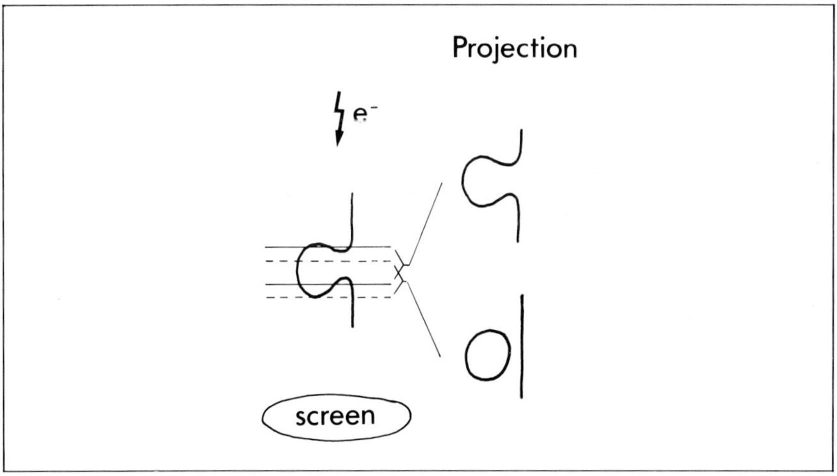

Fig. 2. Schematic representation of a single caveola sectioned with and without the mid-portion of the opening included in a conventional EM thin section (~ 600 Å thick). When the section contains the mid-portion, the projection (image) of an open vesicle is produced. When the section contains only part of the vesicle apparently free profiles may be produced. Reproduced from [14].

half of all connections between individual vesicular units are lost in conventional EM thin sections (500–700 Å thick), with the result that many apparently free vesicular units even represent true single luminal or abluminal open vesicles. This distribution can only be explained by noting that an individual surface connected 'vesicle' must be located exactly at the center of the conventional EM thin section to produce the picture of

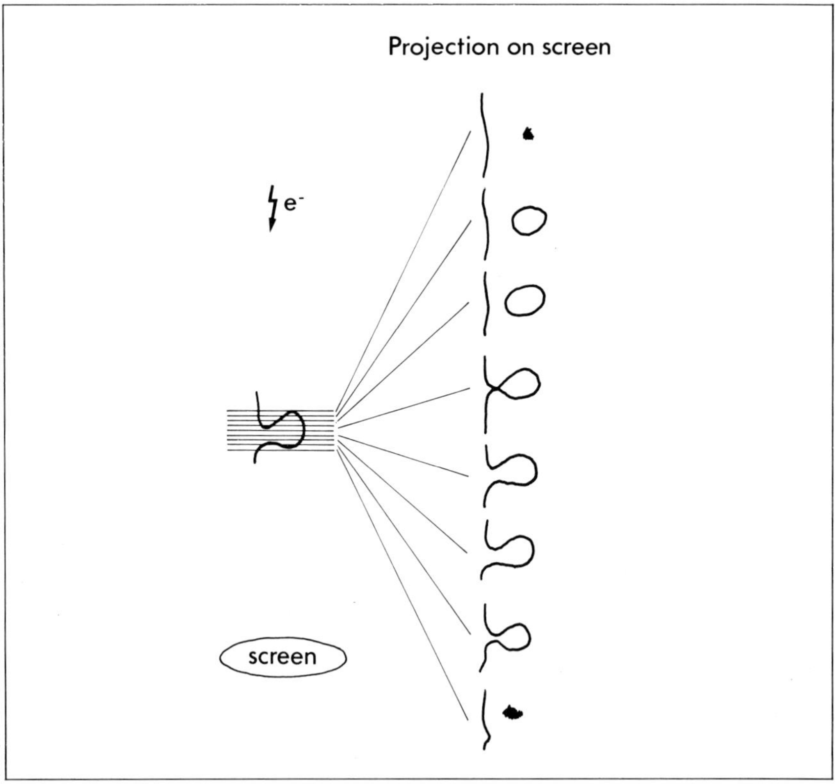

Fig. 3. Tracing of the membrane projections in 7 consecutive ultrathin (~ 140 Å) serial sections of a single surface connected vesicle in frog muscle capillary endothelium. The vesicle first appears as a small electron dense spot in a section that contains only the top of the vesicle. This spot changes into vesicle profiles which grow in size until a maximum is reached, when the vesicle is cut in the mid-portion. Then in the following sections, the vesicle profile decreases and finally disappears in the form of an electron dense spot. The opening to the surface or to another vesicle with which it may be fused, is typically seen on 2–3 of the mid-sections. Depending on how the vesicle is hit by the thin section any degree of opening from fully closed to fully open may be seen. Reproduced from [14].

an open vesicle on the screen. If the vesicle is located slightly off center in the section, the projection of a closed vesicle may be produced (fig. 2). Depending upon the localization of the vesicle within the section, any profile, from fully open (neck diameter ~ 400 Å) to apparently free, may be produced. This is most clearly understood by observing the same vesicle profile in the ultrathin serial sections (figs. 3 and 4). The fact that the many free vesicular profiles in conventional EM sections arise as a result of the EM sectioning, invalidates the use of the localization of tracer molecules in sub-populations of 'vesicles' (luminal, cytoplasmic and abluminal) in single sections to study vesicle involvement in transcapillary exchange of macromolecules. It is important to understand that this limitation applies to any type of fixation with or without prior rapid freezing. It is simply a combination of section thickness and vesicle size and shape. To assure full resolution of vesicle interconnections, it is essential that the thickness of each of the single sections in the series does not exceed 150 Å in analyses of the three-dimensional structure of the plasmalemmal vesicular system. A detailed description of this point is given elsewhere [14].

This three-dimensional organization of the plasmalemmal vesicular system, provided it applies to endothelial cells in vivo, seems incompatible with the original vesicle shuttle hypothesis [27, 28], since this model is based on the notion that a substantial fraction of the apparently free vesicular profiles seen in single conventional EM sections represent truly free entities in the cytoplasm.

Exchange of Macromolecules by Temporary or Permanent Connections between the Two Sets of Plasmalemmal Invaginations

The plasmalemmal vesicular system may still provide a vehicle for transcapillary diffusion of macromolecules if temporary or permanent connections (transendothelial channels) do exist between the luminal and abluminal set of invaginations [12, 14, 15]. This would explain the finding that tracers which are too big to pass the intercellular cleft can be found in the interstitium and in abluminal vesicles some time after injection of the tracers into the bloodstream. It would also explain the time sequence in the labeling of apparent sub-populations of vesicles in conventional EM sections seen in the time tracer studies using small tracers [37, 38, 40]. Fixed at early times after administering the tracer, the tracer would have had time to enter most of the vesicles opening directly to the luminal

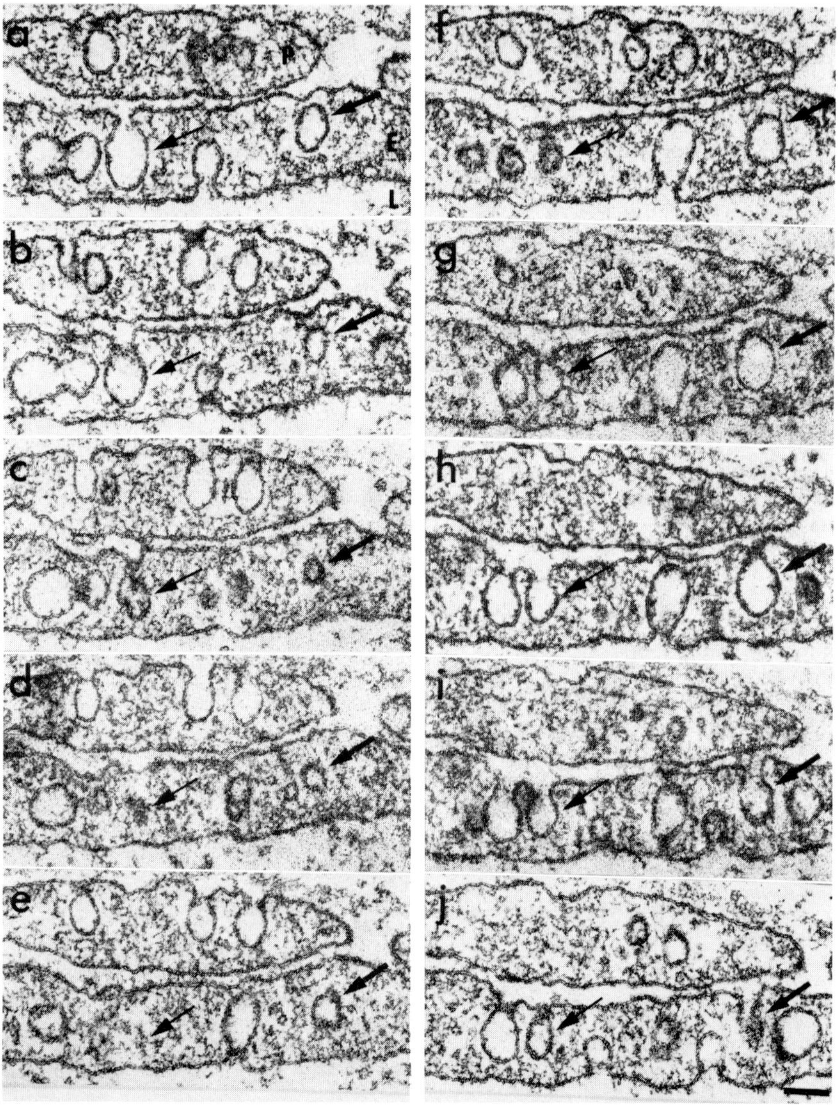

Fig. 4. Ten consecutive ultrathin (~ 140 Å) serial sections of a part of a frog muscle capillary. Note, how vesicles opening directly to the surface can be seen in all configurations between fully open and fully closed, both in the endothelial cell and in the pericyte next to the capillary. Note also, how it is possible to distinguish between two closely located but non-connecting vesicles (thin arrow) and two mutually fused vesicles (wide arrow) from the pattern of appearance and disappearance of the vesicular profiles in consecutive sections. E = endothelium; P = pericyte; L = lumen. Bar = 1000 Å. Reproduced from [14].

surface and a little less than half of the apparently 'cytoplasmic' vesicles, while few abluminal vesicles would be labeled (only those which represent the abluminal end of a channel). Fixed at intermediate times, almost all vesicles belonging to the luminal system would be labeled. An increasing amount of tracer would have diffused through the rare channels and through intercellular junctions and begun to label the abluminal system by retrograde filling. This results in further labeling of 'luminal' vesicles, labeling of a little more than half of the 'cytoplasmic' vesicles, and labeling of an increased number of 'abluminal' vesicles in individual EM thin sections. Fixed at even later times, retrograde filling of the abluminal system proceeds until almost all vesicles become labeled. This is exactly the pattern of labeling which is reported in the studies using heme-peptides and myoglobin [37, 38, 40]. It would also explain the pattern in labeling of 'vesicles' with larger tracers [5, 7, 8, 19, 24, 27, 48]. The difference is that the larger tracers are excluded from the junctional pathway. Furthermore, it is more difficult for the larger tracers to enter the vesicular system due to neck and diaphragm restrictions, thus resulting in an overall lower degree of labeling of all sub-populations of vesicular profiles in individual EM thin sections. The transfer rate depends on the size of the tracer (the larger the molecule, the slower the transfer).

To explain the escape of large dextrans (120 Å diameter) from blood to lymph in dog paw by diffusion [29], only 1 transendothelial channel needs to be open at all times per $\sim$ 500 μm^2 capillary surface area [14] (assuming a channel length of 0.5 µm, an effective open mean channel neck diameter of 200 Å, and a free diffusion coefficient of $0.35 \times 10^{-6}\, cm^2 sec^{-1}$). The value for the fractional 'large pore' area (7×10^{-7}) is close to the value reached by *Renkin and Curry* [30], in a similar calculation based on convective transport at high rates of lymph flow. Based on a separation of diffusion and convection at high and low rates of lymph flow, they argue, however, that the exchange of dextrans can only be explained if about 40% of the flux at low lymph flow rates occurs through a non-hydraulic conductive pathway. This latter view is not shared by other investigators using a similar measuring technique [31; see also *Taylor* et al., this volume].

In our serial reconstructions of the plasmalemmal vesicular system in capillaries from frog mesentery, frog striated muscle and rat heart, we have encountered one transendothelial connection between the luminal and abluminal systems of invaginations [4, 12, 14, 15]. The endothelial volume of these reconstructions covers a total surface area of about 50 μm^2.

In a larger morphometric study on frog mesenteric capillaries using conventional EM techniques [3], we did not encounter any transendothelial channels in capillaries covering a surface area of about 1900 μm^2. Three were found, however, in small venules in a material covering an endothelial surface area of about 500 μm^2 [3]. Thus, transendothelial channels may exist with a frequency which makes them likely candidates for the 'large pores' [17] through which hydrophilic macromolecules may pass the endothelium by diffusion and filtration. I think that this form of involvement of the vesicular system can explain most of the existing data on exchange of macromolecules across non-inflamed capillaries. Apart from explaining the time tracer studies [7, 8, 24, 37, 38, 40], this model also accommodates the important finding that cationized labeled luminal surface membrane does not translocate across the cell to the abluminal cell membrane in conventional EM thin sections [41]. This model is also in good accord with the finding, that there is a gradient in ferritin labeling of the sub-populations of vesicles (luminal, cytoplasmic and abluminal) in conventional EM sections when frog mesenteric capillaries are fixed after various time intervals. 'Luminal' vesicles contain more ferritin particles than 'cytoplasmic' vesicles which in turn contain more particles than 'abluminal' vesicles at all time intervals. This indicates that diffusion is important in exchange of macromolecules [7, 8, 24]. The finding of different microdomains on the endothelium may further contribute to some sorting in the exchange of different types of macromolecules [42].

In view of the very low number of 'large pores' needed to explain blood to lymph transport of macromolecules, other diffusion pathways, such as a few fenestrae or possible focal widenings of intercellular clefts, should also be considered possible candidates. In this case, the plasmalemmal vesicular system may play no role *at all* in transcapillary exchange of macromolecules (see below).

Exchange of Macromolecules by a Combination of Diffusion through Permanent Transendothelial Channels and Series of Fusions and Fissions between Individual Free Cytoplasmic Vesicles

Based on well-timed tracer studies with ferritin in single microvessels from the frog mesentery, *Clough and Michel* have proposed an alternative two-way model for vesicle involvement in transcapillary exchange [7, 8]. Some exchange is believed to occur through permanently open transendothelial channels, and another part through a series of fusions and fissions between free cytoplasmic vesicles. The latter part of the exchange seems incompatible with the three-dimensional organization of the vesicular system as determined by ultrathin serial sectioning of the same type of capillaries [12]. This part is based on the existence of both single vesicles and multi-vesicle units (e.g., units composed of two or more vesicles fused together), as truly free entities in the cytoplasm. The argument which led to the proposal of this model is based on the picture of labeling of the vesicular profiles seen in individual conventional EM thin sections (divided into 'luminal', 'cytoplasmic' and 'abluminal vesicles'), which, as discussed above, is hazardous. The pattern of labeling seen in the individual EM thin sections in these studies is fully compatible with the observed three-dimensional organization of the vesicular system, provided that the two systems of vesicular invaginations make temporary or permanent connections which allow exchange of tracer (see above).

Exchange of Macromolecules by a Combination of Diffusion through Temporary Transendothelial Channels and Vesicle Shuttle between the Two Systems of Invaginations

Based on the previously mentioned finding that cationized labeled luminal membrane does not translocate across the cell to the abluminal membrane, the original vesicle translocation hypothesis has recently been revised [41, 42]. It is now proposed, that macromolecules exchange both via diffusion through transendothelial channels created by temporary fusions between the two systems, and by a revised form of vesicle shuttle. Here, a small separate population of free vesicles shuttle between the two systems of rather permanent vesicle invaginations. Exchange by direct fusion between the two systems of invaginations is called convective transcytosis and the free vesicle shuttle between the two sets of invaginations is called dissipative transcytosis. Both models for transport are compatible with the three-dimensional organization of the vesicular system as analyzed by ultrathin serial sectioning [4, 12, 14, 15]. If both forms of transport mechanisms exist, the relative importance of each remains to be determined.

Exchange of Macromolecules without Involvement of the Vesicular System

Based on the low fraction of truly free cytoplasmic vesicles in combination with the very rare occurrence of transendothelial channels, it is also possible that the plasmalemmal vesicular system plays no role *at all* in transfer of macromolecules across capillary walls. The exchange may, instead, occur via diffusion and filtration through a few gaps, fenestrae or open junctions scattered in the microcirculation. The most important argument against this hypothesis is that open junctions and fenestrae seem confined to venous microvessels [3, 39]. Furthermore, gaps seem to be present only during inflammatory conditions and they too are located mainly in small venous capillaries [43, 13]. It thus becomes difficult to explain the transfer of large tracers across the capillary wall in non-venous parts of the microcirculation during non-inflammatory conditions [7, 8, 40].

The Exact Number of Free Vesicles in Endothelial Cells

The method of ultrathin serial sectioning [12] is the most direct (and most time consuming) approach to determine the true fraction of free vesicles in endothelial cells. Using this method, it is established in different types of endothelial cells [4, 12, 14, 15], that less than 1% of the total population of vesicles are free. This contrasts dramatically to the 50–80% vesicular profiles without apparent communication to the surface seen in conventional EM thin sections.

Estimates may also be based on filling of the vesicular system after fixation with different types of tracers. This method gives the same overall impression, namely, that a large part of the apparently free profiles communicate with the surface [2, 6, 11, 22, 23, 44]. In a study on dog heart capillaries, *Karnovsky and Shea* [22] noted that probably few vesicles were free, based on labeling of previously fixed capillaries with lanthanum. However, the fraction of truly free vesicles is often reported to be higher than 1%. *Chien* et al. [6] estimated that 8% are truly free in arterial endothelium from canine carotid artery, based on labeling of the vesicular system with ruthenium red. In the eel rete mirabile capillaries, a large fraction of vesicular profiles has been reported to represent discrete free vesicles [45]. In lymphatic endothelium *Jones* et al. [20] estimated that 90% of the apparently free vesicles were actually in communication with the cell exterior. In frog perineurial cells, it was found that practically all vesicular profiles connected to the cell surface [36].

How can this discrepancy be explained? First of all, it is questionable whether the tracer can actually penetrate all surface connected vesicles after fixation due to possible restrictions in the diaphragms separating individually fused vesicles. Secondly, endothelial cells also contain smooth endoplasmatic reticulum, which in single cross sections may yield profiles indistinguishable from smooth plasmalemmal vesicular profiles. These estimates will, therefore, inevitably overestimate the number of truly free vesicles. This is of particular importance in special endothelial cells like capillaries from eel rete mirabile, where a special tubular system is well-developed [44]. Since this tubular system yields membrane profiles in the single EM sections that are similar to the plasmalemmal vesicular profiles, it is impossible to determine the true fraction of free plasmalemmal vesicles by tracer labeling in these cells [45].

Recently a new technique using high voltage EM on thick sections was used to estimate the number of truly free vesicles in diaphragm capillaries [*Wagner,* this volume]. The picture is very similar to the reconstruction models from the ultrathin serial sections, except that the fraction of truly free vesicular units (single vesicles or vesicles fused together) is somewhat higher than the fraction found using serial sectioning. Again, it is questionable whether high voltage EM permits sufficient resolution of vesicle interconnections, considering the shape of the vesicles and their close apposition. This criticism is fully understood by observing the close packing of vesicular units in the reconstructed model of a segment of a frog striated muscle capillary (fig. 1). No tilting on this capillary segment would allow a clear determination of true vesicle interconnections. Finally, it is questionable if it is possible to determine whether a vesicular unit is located centrally in the thick section (and thus truly free) or located close to the end of the section where it may connect to another vesicular unit in the next thick section (which is not there). This latter difficulty would be avoided in high voltage EM studies on whole cultured endothelial cells. Apart from the question of what fraction of the vesicles are truly free, the reconstructions emerging from the high voltage electronmicroscopy show a striking similarity to the models constructed from the ultrathin serial sectioning, picturing most of the vesicular units as invaginations from the cell surface.

Fixation Artifacts

The analyses of the three-dimensional organization of the plasmalemmal vesicular system [4, 12, 14, 15] were performed on tissues fixed initially with glutaraldehyde-formaldehyde and postfixed with OsO_4. This procedure was introduced by *Karnovsky* [21]. The glutaraldehyde-formaldehyde mixture has since been the primary fixative of choice in most laboratories because it combines a rapid penetration and immobilization of intracellular structures by formaldehyde, followed by a further stabilizing by the more slowly penetrating glutaraldehyde. The earlier use of OsO_4 as the primary fixative is not recommended, because it may lead to artifactual vesiculations of cell membranes [18].

Some authors argue that vesicles may be predominantly free in vivo, but during fixation, race towards the two cell surfaces where they get stuck [45, 46, see also *Clough,* this volume]. This would explain the three-dimensional organization of the plasmalemmal vesicular system found by ultrathin serial sectioning. The extent to which fixation may affect the three-dimensional organization of the vesicular system should, therefore, be investigated. Almost all studies on vesicle involvement in transcapillary exchange have been performed on fixed tissue. If fixation changes the overall organization of the vesicular system, all earlier data on vesicle involvement in transcapillary exchange of macromolecules would be invalidated. There is evidence which indicates that this does not occur, however. The most direct evidence comes from a numerical study on vesicle profiles connected to the luminal side of frog muscle capillaries containing a high concentration of naturally occuring plasmaproteins [15]. In this study, it was shown that half of the total population of vesicular profiles at the time of fixation contained plasmaproteins in a concentration similar to the concentration in the lumen. The other half of the vesicular profiles, like the interstitium, contained no plasmaproteins. This labeling is exactly complementary to the labeling of vesicular profiles connected to the interstitium in already fixed frog mesenteric capillaries [3]. If fixation induced artifactual fusion of in vivo free vesicles, one would expect a concentration gradient in plasmaproteins between lumen, vesicles opening directly to the lumen and vesicular units opening to the lumen via other vesicles. This was not seen [15]. Furthermore, if the fixation induces significant artifactual fusions between vesicles, it is odd that all multi-vesicle invaginations always open to the surface via *one* open vesicle. One would also expect to find transendothelial channels in high numbers. Finally, smooth plasmalemmal vesicles would be the only intracellular type of vesicles exhibiting this fixation induced fusion since fusions between other vesicles with established transport functions (e.g., coated vesicles, synaptic vesicles, vesicles in multivesicular bodies and hormone granules) do not fuse during fixation. There are reported differences in the distribution of plasmalemmal vesicular profiles in conventional single EM thin sections of glutaraldehyde and rapidly frozen rabbit lung microvessels [25]. However, the fraction of apparently cytoplasmic vesicular profiles in conventional single EM thin sections is greater in glutaraldehyde fixed endothelium than in rapidly frozen endothelium (about 75% versus 62% of the total population of vesicles). This indicates that fixation with glutaraldehyde or rapid freezing may affect the plasmalemmal vesicular system differently. This study contradicts, however, the proposal [45, 46] that in vivo truly free vesicles fuse with the surface membrane or surface connected vesicles during fixation, as this mechanism would result in a dramatic difference in the opposite direction.

Three-Dimensional Organization of the Plasmalemmal Vesicular System in Non-endothelial Cell Types

To determine whether the organization of the vesicular system found in endothelium is peculiar to endothelium alone or is more widespread, I have further analyzed the three-dimensional organization of the vesicular system in mesothelial cells and pericytes by ultrathin serial sectioning.

Mesothelium: 908 vesicular units were followed in 2 series of mesothelium from frog mesentery as described earlier [11]. The series contained 21 and 24 serial sections, each with a thickness of 120–150 Å. The total length of mesothelium was 30 μm and covered a surface area of approx. 10 μm^2. Among the 908 vesicles fully included in the series it was found that only 4 vesicles were possibly free. In individual conventional thin sections of mesothelium, 71% of the vesicles show no connection to the surface (n = 2000). No transmesothelial channels were seen [*Frøkjær-Jensen*, unpublished].

Pericyte: The organization of 104 vesicles in pericytes around two muscle capillaries in 21 and 22 sections was similarly analyzed. Only 1 vesicle was found truly free [15].

These analyses clearly show that the three-dimensional organization found in endothelial cells also applies to other cell types such as mesothelial cells and pericytes. In all three cell types, less than 1% of the total population of vesicles are truly free. It is, therefore, likely that practically all vesicular profiles connect to the surface in 'vesicle' rich cells, where connections between individual vesicle profiles are common in individual EM sections. Similar fusions between other vesicle types with known transport function (e.g., synaptic vesicles, coated vesicles, vesicles in multivesicular bodies) are not normally seen.

Alternative Functions for the Plasmalemmal Vesicular System Non-related to Transcapillary Exchange of Macromolecules

A capillary segment with an endothelial surface area of 1000 μm^2 contains about 125,000 vesicular units, invaginating from the cell surface. In this segment only 2 connections between the two separate sets of vesicular invaginations from the luminal and abluminal surface are needed to explain blood to lymph transport of macromolecules (e.g., dextran, dia. 120 Å) by diffusion and filtration [14, 30]. This disproportion between the number of vesicles and the very rare occurrence of transendothelial channels in itself makes it likely that the plasmalemmal vesicular system serves other more important functions than transcapillary exchange. What, then, are the more basic cell physiological functions of this interesting system, shared by endothelial cells and other cell types rich in vesicular profiles? In recent years, intensive studies on endothelial cells, both on intact capillaries in vivo and on cultured endothelial cells from different vascular segments in vitro, have demonstrated that the endothelial lining of the vascular system throughout the body possesses an astonishing capability for biochemical processing of blood borne substances [32, 9, see also *Ryan,* this volume].

This new insight is very important since it implies that the vascular system can no longer be considered as merely a transport system in which the endothelium just serves a barrier function for proper exchange of gases, water and solutes between blood and tissue. The entire system, on the contrary, must now be regarded as a biochemically highly active 'organ', which may even perform various tasks in different parts of the body.

One immediate function of the plasmalemmal vesicular system is that it increases the surface area by approximately 100%. This, in itself, does not elicit great enthusiasm since the endothelial cell has one of the largest

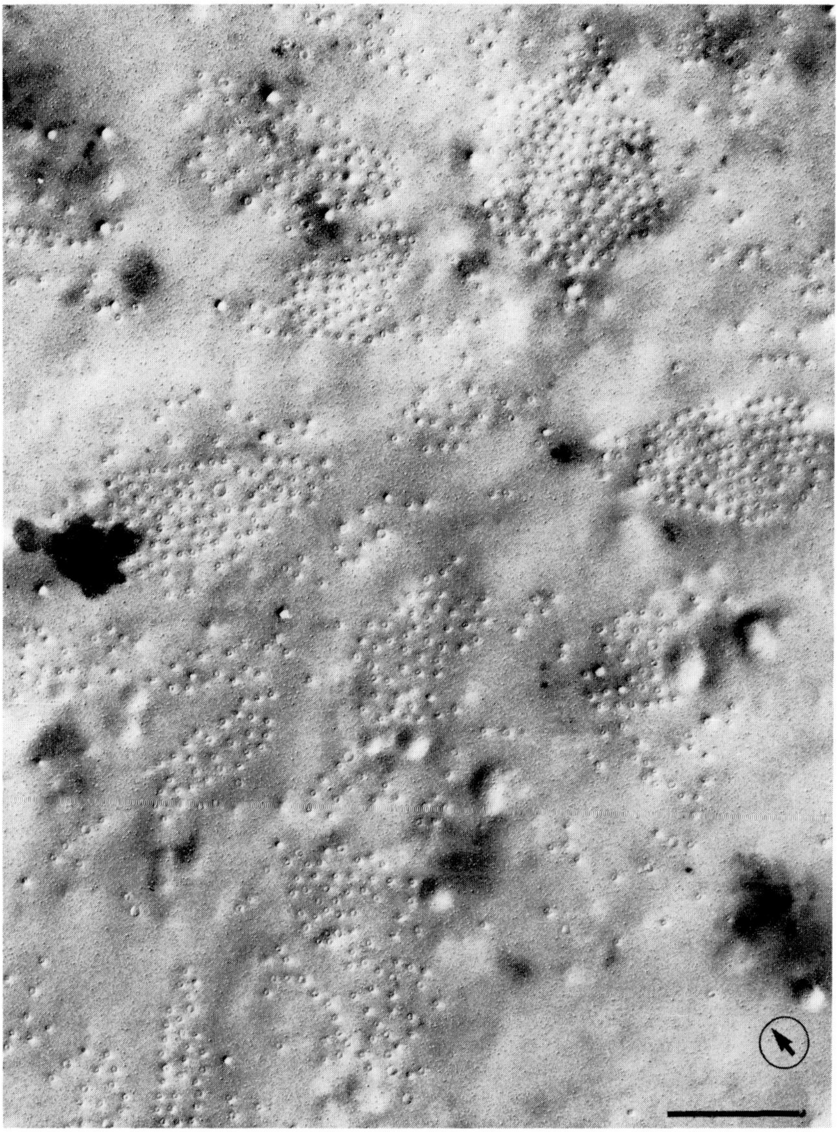

Fig. 5. Surface replica of an endothelial cell from a confluent monolayer culture of a pulmonary artery endothelium. The P-face of the cell surface facing the flask is exposed. The openings of the caveolae are typically organized in patches of closely packed hexagonal arrays. The circled arrow indicates the direction of shadowing. Bar = 1 μm.

surface area to volume ratios of all cell types. Why should it need even more? With the many newly discovered functions of the endothelium, however, one cannot rule out the possibility that endothelial cells, in fact, need all available membrane to accommodate the many enzymes and receptors which perform their various tasks during passage of the blood.

Furthermore, it seems as if the enzymes and the receptors are selectively incorporated in the surface membrane or in the membrane of the plasmalemmal invaginations. Some enzymes, such as ATPase and 5'nucleotidase, appear to reside specifically within the vesicle membrane [32]. Others, such as angiotensin-converting enzyme and carboxy peptidase N, appear to be properties of the plasma membrane including both vesicle membranes and endothelial projections [32]. Carbonic anhydrase exhibits a patchy distribution on the endothelial surface [32] while calmodulin, a specific calcium binding protein, can be found in some, but not all, vesicle membranes [33]. Thus, the plasmalemmal vesicular system may function as a sub-compartment for processing of some specific blood-borne substances.

The vesicular system is not a rigid permanent system. It may change dramatically under various conditions. The number of vesicular profiles was reported to increase 10-fold during gestation in pulmonary capillaries of fetal lambs [35] and the number of 'vesicles' was found to double in lung capillaries and in type I epithelial cells of isolated, perfused dog lungs after acute, severe edema formation [10]. Acute hypertension is also reported to increase the number of vesicular profiles in mammalian brain capillaries [47]. It is most likely that these situations reflect an increase in plasmalemmal invaginations from the cell surface, which in individual conventional EM thin sections is observed as an increase in number of vesicular profiles.

Freeze-fracture studies on endothelial cells in culture show that the vesicular system can change within seconds [16]. In confluent monolayers of endothelial cells cultured from calf pulmonary artery, the vesicular openings (stomata) are frequently seen to occur in hexagonally packed patches or bands, in certain areas (fig. 5). Other areas may be almost devoid of stomata. When confluent monolayers are treated with trypsin and EDTA for 30–60 s, the cells separate from each other, round up and detach from the growth surface. Cells fixed in this situation lose the unevenly distributed but highly ordered patches of stomata from the cell surface. In contrast, multi-vesicle clusters become a prominent feature within the cytoplasm (fig. 6). The few remaining openings to the surface

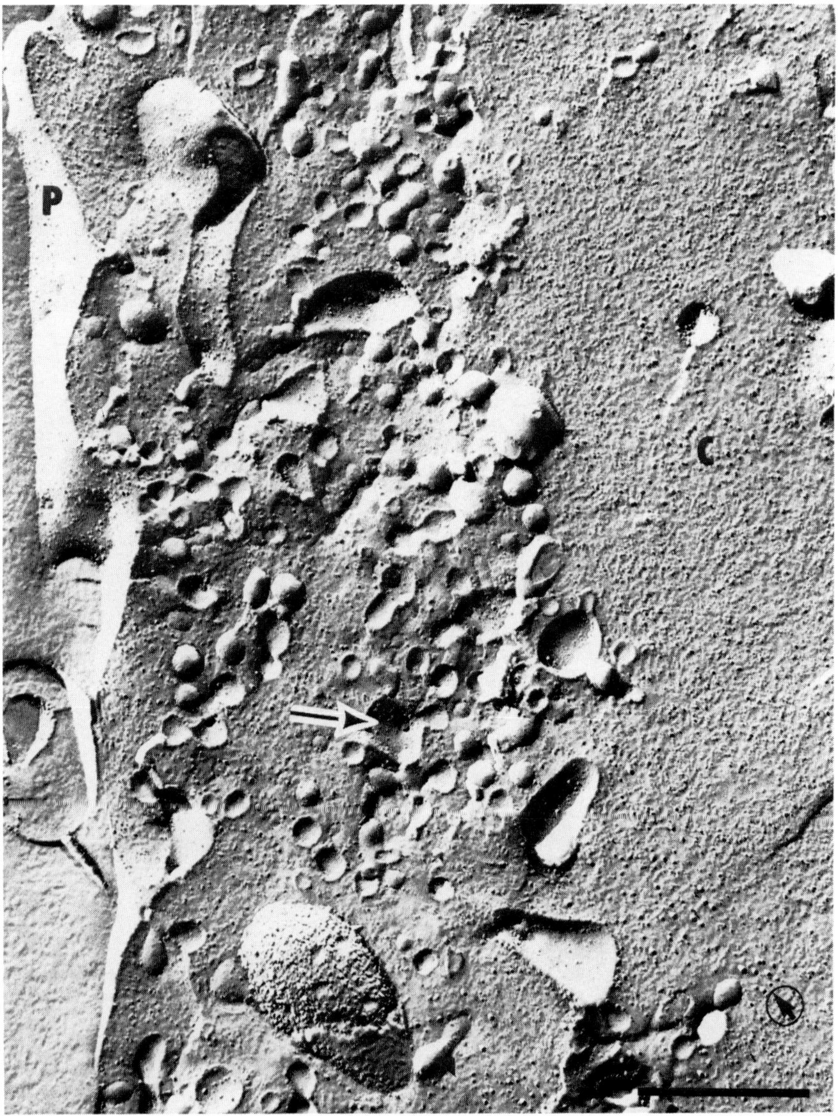

Fig. 6. Replica of a freeze-fractured endothelial cell, rounded up by treatment of a confluent monolayer culture (same culture as used in figure 5) with trypsin and EDTA for 60 s. Multi-vesicle clusters become numerous in the cytoplasm. P = P-face of the surface membrane; C = cytoplasm; white arrow = multi-vesicle cluster. The circled arrow indicates the direction of shadowing. Bar = 0.5 μm. Reproduced from [34].

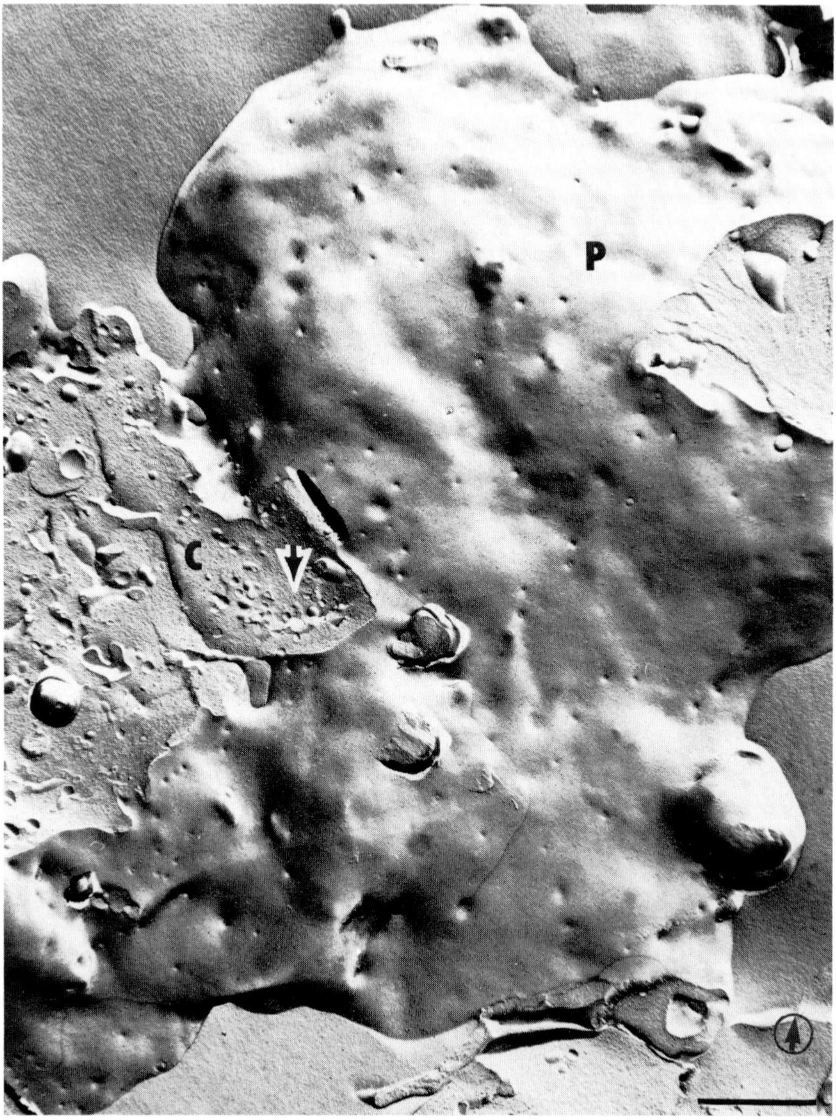

Fig. 7. Surface replica of a freeze-fractured endothelial cell, rounded up by treatment of a confluent monolayer (same culture as used for figs. 5 and 6) with trypsin and EDTA for 60 s. P-face of the cell surface is exposed. The ordered arrays of vesicle openings to the surface seen in fig. 5 have disappeared. The remaining openings are scattered more evenly throughout the whole cell surface. C = cytoplasm; white arrow = multi-vesicle cluster in the cell interior. The circled arrow indicates the direction of shadowing. Bar = 1 μm.

become more evenly distributed (fig. 7). This we take as an indication that the cellular rounding-up in response to treatment with trypsin/EDTA is accompanied by infolding of the surface membrane areas which contained the highly ordered patches and bands of stomata. It is still unsettled whether the multi-vesicle clusters all remain connected to the surface via the reduced number of surface openings or if they are truly internalized. In either case the observation shows that the organization of the plasmalemmal vesicular system can undergo rapid changes. The infolding/ internalization of the membrane may serve to preserve plasma membrane during changes in cell shape and/or may be a mechanism to protect enzymes and receptors located in the plasma membrane during a cellular response to injurious substances (a membrane – enzyme / receptor storage – function). In fact, the finding that endothelial cells which round up in response to mechanical disturbance or cold shock do not exhibit the same dramatic loss of ordered openings to the surface [*Frøkjær-Jensen and Ryan,* unpublished] would favor the latter explanation.

Summary

Analyses of the three-dimensional organization of the plasmalemmal vesicular system by ultrathin (~ 140 Å) serial sectioning of endothelial cells from frog mesenteric [12], frog striated muscle [14, 15] and rat heart capillaries [4] have shown that truly free cytoplasmic vesicles are extremely rare. Instead, the many apparently free vesicle profiles seen in conventional EM sections are components of two separate sets of invaginations of the cell surfaces; one set communicates with the lumen, the other set with the abluminal side of the capillary wall. The same organization of the plasmalemmal vesicular system is also demonstrated in non-endothelial cells such as mesothelial cells from frog mesentery and in pericytes around muscle capillaries. The implication of this organization for current models for transcapillary exchange of hydrophilic macromolecules is discussed. If the vesicular system (as a side-function) is involved in exchange of macromolecules across the capillary wall this transport is most likely to occur by diffusion and filtration through rare temporary or permanent connections between the luminal and abluminal set of vesicular invaginations. Freeze-fracture studies of cultured endothelial cells show that the plasmalemmal vesicular system can change dramatically within seconds during changes in cell shape. In addition, endothelial cells contain a vast number of caveolae and vesicular invaginations in comparison with the rare occurrence of transendothelial channels. Together, these facts suggest that the plasmalemmal vesicular system in endothelial cells, like in other 'vesicle'-rich cells serves more basic cell physiological functions than transcapillary exchange of macromolecules. It may serve as a membrane bank during changes in cell shape and/or serve to store membrane bound enzymes and receptors, which may be exposed directly on the cell surface or hidden in the plasmalemmal vesicular system, depending on cellular needs.

Acknowledgments

Part of this work was carried out while the author was visiting the Department of Medicine (D–58), University of Miami, USA. I wish to thank Professor *Una S. Ryan* for a very stimulating year in her laboratory and for a critical review of the manuscript. Dr. *Mike Brown* is thanked for linguistic help as well as for the loan of his Macintosh computer. The author holds an established Niels Bohr Investigatorship, sponsored by Egmont H. Petersens Foundation, under the Royal Danish Academy of Sciences and Letters. The work was further supported in part by grants from The Council for Tobacco Research – USA, Inc., from NATO and from Weimanns Foundation.

References

1 Bundgaard, M.: Evidence for tortuous pathways accessible to macromolecules through the junctional region of capillary endothelium. J. Physiol., Lond. *345:* 42P (1983).

2 Bundgaard, M.; Frøkjær-Jensen, J.; Crone, C.: Endothelial plasmalemmal vesicular profiles as elements in a system of branching invaginations from the cell surface. Proc. natn. Acad. Sci. USA *76:* 6439-6442 (1979).

3 Bundgaard, M.; Frøkjær-Jensen, J.: Functional aspects of the ultrastructure of terminal blood vessels: A quantitative study on consecutive segments of the frog mesenteric microvasculature. Microvasc. Res. *23:* 1–30 (1982).

4 Bundgaard, M.; Hagman, P.; Crone, C.: The three-dimensional organization of plasmalemmal vesicular profiles in the endothelium of rat heart capillaries. Microvasc. Res. *25:* 358–368 (1983).

5 Bruns, R. R.; Palade, G. E.: Studies on blood capillaries. II. Transport of ferritin molecules across the wall of muscle capillaries. J. Cell Biol. *37:* 277–299 (1968).

6 Chien, S.; Laufer, L.; Handley, D. A.: Vesicle distribution in the arterial endothelium determined with ruthenium red as an extracellular marker. J. Ultrastruct. Res. *79:* 198–206 (1982).

7 Clough, G.; Michel, C. C.: The role of vesicles in the transport of ferritin through frog endothelium. J. Physiol., Lond. *315:* 127–142 (1981).

8 Clough, G.: The steady-state transport of cationized ferritin by endothelial cell vesicles. J. Physiol., Lond. *328:* 389–401 (1982).

9 Crone, C.: The function of capillaries; in Baker (ed.), Recent Advances in Physiology no. 10, pp. 125–162 (Churchill Livingstone, London 1984).

10 De Fouw, D. O.; Chinard, F. P.: Variation in cellular attenuation and vesicle numerical densities in capillary endothelium and type I epithelium of isolated, perfused dog lungs after acute severe edema formation. Microvasc. Res. *26:* 15–26 (1983).

11 Frøkjær-Jensen, J.; Bundgaard, M.: Sessile vesicle "clusters" in frog mesenteric capillaries. A new concept of vesicular organization in the endothelial cell. Microvasc. Res. *18:* 297 (1979).

12 Frøkjær-Jensen, J.: Three-dimensional organization of plasmalemmal vesicles in endothelial cells. An analysis by serial sectioning of frog mesenteric capillaries. J. Ultrastruct. Res. *73:* 9–20 (1980).

13 Frøkjær-Jensen, J.: Permeability of single muscle capillaries to potassium ions. Microvasc. Res. *24:* 168–183 (1982).

14 Frøkjær-Jensen, J.: The plasmalemmal vesicular system in capillary endothelium. Conventional electron microscopic (EM) thin sections compared with the picture arising from ultrathin (~ 140 Å) serial sectioning; in Messmer, Hammersen (eds.), Structure and function of endothelial cells, Prog. appl. Microcirc., vol. 1, pp. 17–34 (Karger, Basel 1983).

15 Frøkjær-Jensen, J.: The plasmalemmal vesicular system in striated muscle capillaries and in pericytes. Tissue & Cell. *16:* 31–42 (1984).

16 Frøkjær-Jensen, J.; Ryan, U. S.: Reorganization of the plasmalemmal vesicular system during shape changes of endothelial cells in cultures. Int. J. Microcirc. Clin. Exp. *3*: 362 (1984).

17 Grotte, G.: Passage of dextran molecules across the blood lymph barrier. Acta chir. scand. (suppl.) *221:* 1–84 (1956).

18 Hayat, M. A.: Fixation for Electronmicroscopy (Acad. Press, New York 1981).

19 Jennings, M. A.; Florey, H.: An investigation of some properties of endothelium related to capillary permeability. Proc. Roy. Soc. Ser. B. *167:* 39–63 (1967).

20 Jones, W. R.; O'Morchoe, P. J.; O'Morchoe, C. C.: The organization of endocytotic vesicles in lymphatic endothelium. Microvasc. Res. *25:* 286–299 (1983).

21 Karnovsky, M. J.: The ultrastructural basis of capillary permeability studied with peroxidase as a tracer. J. Cell Biol. *35:* 213–236 (1967).

22 Karnovsky, M. J.; Shea, A. M.: Transcapillary transport by pinocytosis. Microvasc. Res. *2:* 353–360 (1970).

23 Kobayashi, S.: Ferritin labelling in the fixed muscle capillary. A doubt on the tracer-experiments as the basis for the vesicular transport theory. Arch. histol. Jap. *32:* 81–86 (1970).

24 Loudon, M. F.; Michel, C. C.; White, I. F.: The labelling of vesicles in frog endothelial cells with ferritin. J. Physiol., Lond. *296:* 97–112 (1979).

25 Mazzone, R. W.; Kornblau, S. M.: Pinocytotic vesicles in the endothelium of rapidly frozen rabbit lung. Microvasc. Res. *21:* 193–211 (1981).

26 Palade, G. E.: Fine structure of blood vessels. J. appl. Physics *24:* 1424 (1953).

27 Palade, G. E.: Blood capillaries of the heart and other organs. Circulation *24:* 368–384 (1961).

28 Palade, G. E.; Bruns, R. R.: Structural modulations of plasmalemmal vesicles. J. Cell Biol. *37:* 633–653 (1968).

29 Renkin, E. M.: Relation of capillary morphology to transport of fluid and large molecules: A review. Acta physiol. scand. (suppl.) *463:* 81–91 (1979).

30 Renkin, E. M.; Curry, F. E.: Endothelial permeability: Pathways and modulations; in Fishman (ed.), Endothelium, pp. 248–259 (New York Acad. Sci. Series 1982).

31 Rutili, G.; Granger, D. N.; Taylor, A. E.; Parker, J. C.; Mortillaro, N. A.: Analysis of lymphatic protein data. IV. Comparison of the different methods used to estimate reflection coefficients and permeability-surface area products. Microvasc. Res. *23:* 347–360 (1982).

32 Ryan, U. S.: Structural bases for metabolic activity. Ann. Rev. Physiol. *44:* 223–239 (1982).

33 Ryan, U. S.; Ryan, J. W.: Surface properties of pulmonary endothelial cells. In: Sur-

face phenomena in hemorheology; their theoretical, experimental and clinical aspects. Ann. N.Y. Acad. Sci. *416:* 441–456 (1983).

34 Ryan, U. S.; Frøkjær-Jensen, J.: Pulmonary endothelium and processing of plasma solutes: Structure and function; in Said (ed.), Pulmonary circulation and pulmonary vascular injury. (Futura Publications, New York 1985.)

35 Schneeberger, E. E.: Plasmalemmal vesicles in pulmonary capillary endothelium of developing fetal lamb lungs. Microvasc. Res. *25:* 40–55 (1983).

36 Shinowara, N. L.; Michel, M. E.; Rapoport, S. I.: Morphological correlates of permeability in the frog perineurium: Vesicles and 'transcellular channels'. Cell Tissue Res. *227:* 11–22 (1982).

37 Simionescu, N.; Simionescu, M.; Palade, G. E.: Permeability of muscle capillaries to exogenous myoglobin. J. Cell Biol. *57:* 424–452 (1973).

38 Simionescu, N.; Simionescu, M.; Palade, G. E.: Permeability of muscle capillaries to small heme-peptides. Evidence for the existence of patent transendothelial channels. J. Cell Biol. *64:* 586–607 (1975).

39 Simionescu, N.; Simionescu, M.; Palade, G. E.: Open junctions in the endothelium of the postcapillary venules of the diaphragm. J. Cell Biol. *79:* 27–44 (1978 a).

40 Simionescu, N.; Simionescu, M.; Palade, G. E.: Structural basis of permeability in sequential segments of the microvasculature of the diaphragm. II. Pathway followed by microperoxidase across the endothelium. Microvasc. Res. *15:* 17–36 (1978 b).

41 Simionescu, N.; Simionescu, M.: Hydrophilic pathways of capillary endothelium, a dynamic system; in Ussing, Bindslev, Lassen, Sten-Knudsen (eds.), Alfred Benzon Symposium 15, Water transport across epithelia, pp. 228–247 (Munksgaard, Copenhagen 1981).

42 Simionescu, N.: Cellular aspects of transcapillary exchange. Physiol. Rev. *63:* 1536–1579 (1983).

43 Svensjö, E.; Arfors, K.-E.; Grega, G. J.: Morphological and physiological correlation of bradykinin-induced macromolecular efflux. Am. J. Physiol. C. *236:* H600–H606 (1979).

44 Rasio, E. A.; Bendayan, M.; Goresky, C. A.: The effect of hyperosmolarity on the permeability and structure of the capillaries of the isolated Rete mirabile of the eel. Circulation Res. *49:* 661–676 (1981).

45 Wagner, R. C.; Robinson, C. S.: Tannic acid analysis of permeability pathways in the capillaries of the rete mirabile: Demonstration of the discreteness of endothelial vesicles. J. Ultrastruct. Res. *81:* 37–46 (1982).

46 Wagner, R. C.; Casley-Smith, J. R.: Endothelial vesicles. Microvasc. Res. *21:* 267–298 (1981).

47 Westergaard, E.; Van Deurs, B.; Brøndsted, H. E.: Increased vesicular transfer of horseradish peroxidase across cerebral endothelium, evoked by acute hypertension. Acta neuropath. *35:* 141–152 (1977).

48 Wissig, S. L.: Identification of the small pore in muscle capillaries. Acta physiol. scand. (suppl.) *463:* 33–44 (1979).

J. Frøkjær-Jensen, PhD, Institute of Medical Physiology, Department A, The Panum Institute, University of Copenhagen, Blegdamsvej 3C, DK-2200 Copenhagen (Denmark)

Prog. appl. Microcirc., vol. 9, pp. 43–50 (Karger, Basel 1985)

Discussion of the Presentations: *Wagner, Casley-Smith, Frøkjær-Jensen*

HAMMERSEN: Let us discuss first how fixation procedures, either freezing or chemical, might influence what one sees in super-ultrathin sections, and compare this with those techniques as used by Drs. WAGNER and CASLEY-SMITH. After this initial discussion of vesicle configuration, we can then address the question of vesicular functions including transport.

FRØKJÆR-JENSEN (showed slides): I would like to summarize some arguments against the proposal that vesicles are free. It appears peculiar to me that the sticking together of vesicles and to the cell membranes is a fixation artefact, because the ordered array, which we found in cultured cells, does not support this assumption. The other thing ist that one should find many more transendothelial channels, because why should a vesicle only stick to one of the surfaces which are only a small distance apart. They should sometimes stick to both surfaces, thereby forming transendothelial channels, but we had a hard time to find these.

The next point is that the data of *Mazzone and Kornblau* vary with CASLEY-SMITH's data. They found fewer surface-connected vesicular profiles in conventional EM sections of pulmonary capillaries, which are chemically fixed vs. capillaries that are rapidly frozen.

The final point is that plasmalemmal vesicles would be the only intracellular type of vesicle which would exhibit this type of fixation-induced fusion. All other vesicles that have transport functions never fuse. This is true for coated vesicles, synaptic vesicles, vesicles in multivesicular bodies and hormone granules.

WAGNER: The last point is somewhat misleading, because for some of these other organelles that you are talking about, the spatial separation between them is much greater. They are not closely packed. It seems as though you are putting some credence on cells in tissue culture as being good models in terms of looking at vesicular function. Is that not correct?

FRØKJÆR-JENSEN: Not for macromolecular transport, but I think that cultured EC are a very good system, especially since you can change the system and look at what happens to the vesicles.

WAGNER: There is a system in which fixation artefacts are not a factor, in which vesicular transport can be measured in living cells, and that is the one that I have been using in isolated capillaries. We see uptake here that exhibits kinetics similar to endocytosis. There is sequestration into these vesicles. The inability to elute this internalized label from these cells is evidence to me that this is true sequestration. I would like you to address this question.

FRØKJÆR-JENSEN: I have no doubt at all that vesicular uptake into the cell occurs as a simple cell function.

WAGNER: The obvious experiment is to do exactly the same kind of analysis as you have done in collapsed blood vessels vs. those which have a normal ambient hydrostatic pressure.

FRØKJÆR-JENSEN: That is not so easy.

WAGNER: The prediction would be, that in collapsed vessels you would detect many more internalized vesicles. In fact, if they function as a membrane bank, as you say they do, then they should be greatly increased in collapsed vessels.

FRØKJÆR-JENSEN: I have a question for you. In the first part of your talk, you mentioned that tannic acid was not able to enter all the vesicles in your system, so you used glutaraldehyde. You also used glutaraldehyde in your thick sections, and you also used tannic acid. How is that you see all the vesicles which are free?

WAGNER: I made no claim as to the number or incidence, because too many of the profiles were obscured. However, they were easy to detect. I did not have to look far to find them.

FRØKJÆR-JENSEN: This is a point raised by J. J. FRIEDMAN. Do you really think it is possible to decide if a vesicle, as you showed in the three-dimensional pictures, is located in the middle of a section or close to one of its surfaces?

WAGNER: Yes, if you use reference points above and below that particular structure, as I tried to point out.

WILLIAMSON: I have two comments. My own impression is that the quality of presentation in the frozen tissue hardly warrants the conclusion that Dr. FRØKJÆR-JENSEN's tissue is poorly fixed. The quality of presentation of structure is obviously much superior. Second, in relation to the point that glutaraldehyde fixation may be causing vesicle formation as an artefact. This would be contrary to an early observation when glutaraldehyde was first introduced as a fixative. These were studies in the adrenal cortex, the cells of which displayed many vesicles in the cytoplasm after fixation with osmium. If, however, glutaraldehyde fixation was used these vesicles disappeared. So one had just the opposite effect of what is proposed here as an artefact of glutaraldehyde.

WAGNER: I don't think anybody is saying that the vesicles disappear. I think that all we are talking about are the connections between them.

WILLIAMSON: You are talking about free vesicles vs. vesicular clusters.

CASLEY-SMITH: Can I answer these two points? When I said poor fixation, I didn't mean what an electron-microscopist looking at beautiful pictures normally means when saying: fixation is poor; because, e.g., mitochondria are blown up etc. What I meant was that there exists a very subtle change in excessive duration of fixation with glutaraldehyde. The pictures look good, but I believe that the excessive cross-linking, which is a characteristic feature of glutaraldehyde, can cause vesicles to fuse, when they weren't fused earlier. People fixing for only 30–60 min tend to find free vesicles with tannic acid whereas people fixing for 15–20 h do not. I'm not talking about causation of vesicles by a fixative, not that sort of gross artefact. It's a very fine artefact, which I think can only be revealed by the tannic acid stain. This is only a suggestion that would explain two pieces of contradictory evidence.

U. RYAN: I think we're getting hung-up on the wrong issue here. I would like to ask the first two speakers how they get from their data to their conclusions.

For Dr. WAGNER: What you have shown with the three-dimensional study is, that a variety of configurations of the vesicles exists on the two sides. Since you picked an endothelial cell that has a small luminal to abluminal distance, there is confusion in the middle. That would not be so if you picked a cultured cell or a flatter one. However, regardless of whether any of the vesicles are free or what the fixation step is, the question is: are the vesicles associated with one or the other front or are they wandering around in the middle? I don't see that you presented any evidence that they traverse the cell.

WAGNER: I don't remember making that claim, at least derived from the data.

U. RYAN: You don't make it then. All I want to establish is that you simply showed configurations of vesicles on one or the other surface. Is that all what we can conclude?

WAGNER: No, I presented what I believe to be single and compound vesicular structures completely free.

U. RYAN (for CASLEY-SMITH): You analyzed your data by categorizing the vesicles as in fusion-mode or in fission-mode. I don't understand how either of you can make the assumption that they are going in and out or going across the cell.

CASLEY-SMITH: My categorization, and this is on conventional sections, of the fusion- or fission-mode was following the classification of *Palade and Bruns*.

U. RYAN: But do either of you have any functional evidence that this is happening?

CASLEY-SMITH: If you accept the functional evidence of vesicular transport, then it seems worthwhile using these categories of fission- and fusion-mode. The point is that there is a considerable difference between the proportions found in these two modes, between chemical fixation and freezing. The reason is that the chemical fixation is slow and allows vesicles to pass from the fusion-mode to the fission-mode, when they would normally disappear, but they can't.

WAUGH: There isn't any doubt that in the thin sections there aren't any free vesicles in those specimens, and the central question is whether or not free vesicles exist in the freeze material or whether they disappear during the fixation process. One of the ways that you can look at this argument is to think about the mechanisms of what should happen during the fusion process. What is the composition of these vesicular surfaces? Are they protein? Is there some kind of cytoskeleton associated with these structures or is it possibly a simple lipid bilayer?

WAGNER: These are lipoprotein membranes. There are no coated portions of these nude vesicles.

WAUGH: If there is a significant amount of protein in these membranes, as they are fixed in glutaraldehyde, it is going to become less and less likely that you are going to be able to have fusion, because you have to deform the surfaces in order for the vesicles to fuse. So as they become more rigid during the fixation process, it's going to be harder and harder to deform them, to complete the fusion process.

SHEA: I would like to draw attention to a paper by *McGuire* that appeared last year using freezing with the slammer, in which he found that the number of caveolae was halved as compared to chemical fixation. That doesn't explain where the structures went to, if they went anywhere, but it is perhaps relevant to the rest of the discussion.

SCHNEEBERGER: The *Mazzone- and Kornblau*-technique was simply spraying Freon onto the lungs, and I think that this is inferior because the rate of freezing is much slower than by doing it with the slammer technique. In terms of composition of the vesicle membrane, we have very nice freeze-fracture evidence that these are not simply phospholipid structures. There are proteins in them and these proteins would become cross-linked by glutaraldehyde fixation and I think we must keep that in mind.

WAGNER: They could be cross-linked between the vesicles as well as within the plane of the membrane.

SCHNEEBERGER: Right. The proteins could conceivably still move within the plane of the lipid bilayer and allow for areas of fusion as Dr. CASLEY-SMITH has suggested.

SILBERBERG: What struck me very much was the symmetry between the two sides of the cells. The luminal side of the cell is under quite different mechanical conditions in the living system than the abluminal side and the fact that you get no difference suggests to me, at any rate, that we are looking at an artefact. What I want to stress is that when you have an invagination, which is the sort of thing I would expect could arise on the luminal side; the time at which this break up into droplets is of the order of between one-thousandth and one-hundredth of a second. So that no fixation process that has been discussed today could actually catch an invagination intact, once the mechanical forces that are producing it have stopped.

CASLEY-SMITH: I think you'll find that freezing, if it crosses an endothelial cell in 0.2 s, might just catch it.

SILBERBERG: Occasionally, yes.

CASLEY-SMITH: It should, because of the distance. One-tenth of a second should cover it.

FRIEDMAN: It occurs to me that until someone has serially sectioned material of short fixation time to determine whether or not there are interrelationships between vesicles, all the rest of the arguments we've heard are entirely specious. You can theorize as much as you like, you can do the calculations as much as you like, there is nothing better than hard data. If it's an artefact then it will show up as an artefact in the serial sections. If it's not then at least we have some tangible information with which to make realistic comparisons.

WAYLAND: I believe that it is quite possible, with modern mathematical reconstruction techniques, to deconvolute a series of pictures taken in the three-dimensional mode that Dr. WAGNER talks about. Thereby achieving a really good three-dimensional picture, not just what we see with the eye, but really to unscramble it. I believe that this is a far more valuable way to go than to having to make millions of serial thin sections, because I think the information is going to be incomplete. Furthermore, I think that this must be studied as a function of rapid freezing, as a function of different fixations and not just stick to some technique in one laboratory and to another in another laboratory.

FRØKJÆR-JENSEN: I actually don't think you will be able to resolve these structural details even with any videotape method, because you have just the various shapes of the vesicle depending upon whether you have a neck of about 400 Å, or the rest of the vesicle which is about 900 Å. How would you resolve that?

WAYLAND: How do you resolve a tumor only a millimeter in diameter in the brain with a beam of X-rays going through the brain? You can do it. It takes very sophisticated mathematics, but it is possible.

CRONE: I want to clarify where we stand with this discussion. As I feel the audience here is convinced that when you do reconstructions of ultrathin serial sections you find that most of the vesicles communicate with either surface. What we have to discuss now is whether this is an artefact or not? Nobody here seems to doubt that we would obtain the same pictures if we took, e.g., *Palade*'s sections and studied them three-dimensionally. Then I have a question to Dr. CASLEY-SMITH: When we count what is, in the literature, called free vesicles in normal thin sections, we find numbers very close to what everybody finds and you confused us by stating otherwise. The only way to find few free vesicles is the cumbersome way of three-dimensional reconstruction and this makes the important difference. Everybody must realize the following: if we prepare ordinary thin sections with the same techniques as used by most others, we have exactly the same results as they have. The non-existence of 'free' vesicles is something which comes via another argument, namely the stacking of ultrathin sections upon each other and searching for the pathways.

CASLEY-SMITH: I should have made that point more clear. You do ultrathin serial sections and the rest of us are too scared to try it. But you have always used 15–20 h glutaraldehyde fixation and it may be that this is the cause why you find no free vesicles and others do.

WAGNER: I would like somebody from the Copenhagen group to explain to us just exactly what the sample size of these small serial section reconstructions is. Are we talking about one series of sections or two or five or ten?

BUNDGAARD: We have reconstructed about ten cubic micrometers of endothelium, containing about two thousand vesicular units.

WAGNER: How many vessels are we talking about?

BUNDGAARD: The reconstructions come from five rat heart capillaries, from mesentery and two series of muscle capillaries.

WILLIAMSON: One important point we have to clear up. Dr. CRONE said that they find the same result in terms of numbers of free vesicles when they fix for 20–25 h and they only find the difference when they do serial reconstructions. Dr. CASLEY-SMITH I think glossed that over. Then the duration of fixation is beside the point here.

CASLEY-SMITH: Yes, and I agree that it would be, except that you can understand that if you have a conventional section, then vesicles which were in fact fused could appear free. I quite agree that the conventional section is not the right way to decide if the vesicle is free or not. But, if there is a fixation artefact from glutaraldehyde, then a very thin ultrathin section of very long fixed material will reveal fused vesicles. Ultrathin sections of a short fixation time will reveal free ones. So far the ultrathin sectioning of a short fixation time has not been performed.

ELMAURO: I hesitate to bring in another variable, but we have looked at the lymphatic endothelium and stained it with tannic acid and ruthenium red. We haven't done thin serial sectioning and again in conventional thin sections we find about 50% of the vesicles appear to be free. But with tannic acid and ruthenium red this percentage is reduced to about 11%, indicating that they are continuous in one way or another with either surface. We also do not find any transendothelial channels. So the vesicles do appear in that short fixation time in lymphatic endothelium to coalesce or to be connected to either surface.

HARALDSSON: Together with Dr. JOHANNSON (Dept. of Anatomy) I have performed experiments in support of the data of Dr. FRØKJÆR-JENSEN. We perfused the isolated rat hindquarter with serum and measured capillary filtration coefficient (CFC) and diffusion capacity for Vitamin B12 together with albumin clearance. Then the hindquarters were fixed by vascular perfusion and we switched back to serum perfusion. Immediately before and after fixation we used protein-free solutions and measured CFC, PS and albumin clearance again and all were reduced in parallel. Both PS for small solutes (vitamin B12), CFC and albumin clearance fell to approximately 50% in support of the suggestion that vesicular transport is not a significant function for albumin transport during normal conditions.

WAGNER: Is that native albumin that you used?

HARALDSSON: Yes.

WAGNER: We have evidence that vesicles specifically exclude native albumin.

HARALDSSON: Ferritin does not exist in the circulation. You have albumin there.

HAMMERSEN: This brings us to the problem of vesicle functions, which we should discuss after having heard the next contributions.

END OF DISCUSSION

Prog. appl. Microcirc., vol. 9, pp. 51–58 (Karger, Basel 1985)

Quantitative Transport of Macromolecules by Endothelial Cell Vesicles

G. Clough, C. C. Michel

Department of Physiology and Biophysics, St. Mary's Hospital Medical School, London, and
University Laboratory of Physiology, University of Oxford, Oxford, England

Introduction

Over the past few years there has been increasing scepticism concerning the contribution of endothelial cell vesicles to vascular permeability [7]. We have tried to estimate this contribution by examining the time sequence and pattern of labelling of the endothelial cell vesicles of frog mesenteric capillaries after exposure of the luminal cell surface of the endothelium (and hence the luminal vesicles) to the macromolecule ferritin.

We believe that these studies have shed some light on the role endothelial cell vesicles play in macromolecular transport, and have also helped us to examine the question as to whether vesicles are indeed artifacts of the procedures used to investigate them.

Material and Methods

In all our studies we have used a modification of the single vessel perfusion technique combined with a morphological study of the perfused vessel [2–4]. In this way we are able to obtain a quantitative description of the time course of labelling of the vesicle system with a tracer, when the physiological conditions of the vessel are carefully monitored and the fixation procedures accurately controlled.

Briefly, single capillaries of the exteriorised mesentery of decerebrated frogs are cannulated with a sharpened glass micropipette (tip diameter: 10–15 μm) filled with a solution containing measured amounts of the electron dense tracer ferritin (a_{es} = 6 nm). The pressure in the pipette was held at 0 cm H_2O during cannulation and then raised abruptly to 30 cm H_2O and the vessel perfused with ferritin solution for a carefully recorded period. The temperature of the perfusate and the tissue was controlled by controlling the temperature of the frog Ringer solution irrigating the exteriorised mesentery.

In one series of experiments, the perfused capillaries were initially fixed by flooding the whole tissue with 2% osmium tetroxide at recorded times after the commencement of perfusion of the vessel. In the second series, 6% glutaraldehyde was used as the primary fixative. Tissues from all experiments were then immersed in 6% glutaraldehyde for 4 to 12 h.

All the vessels were prepared routinely for electron microscopy, and thin (50 nm) transverse sections of the perfused vessels examined using transmission electron microscopy. Endothelial cell thickness was estimated from photographs of the endothelium at a magnification of 87,000 × and mean vesicle diameter calculated from two perpendicular measurements of the internal diameter of each vesicle.

Classification of Vesicles

Vesicles were divided into three populations; luminal and abluminal vesicles are the caveolae which open by a short neck to the blood and tissue surfaces of the endothelium, respectively; cytoplasmic vesicles are those which appear to lie wholly within the cell cytoplasm. The labelling of vesicles with molecules of ferritin is defined as N_L/N_T; the number of vesicles in any population (N_L) containing one or more ferritin molecules expressed as a fraction of the total number of vesicles counted in that population (N_T), and also as F/N_L; the number of ferritin molecules (F) within any labelled vesicle. All these estimates were corrected for sectioning losses and their 95% confidence limits calculated [3–5].

Results and Discussion

We have described the distribution and labelling of endothelial cell vesicles of the frog mesentery with molecules of ferritin under various physiological conditions and these data can be found in detail elsewhere [2–5].

Four important general observations can be made concerning these data:

(1) We have demonstrated that when single capillaries are perfused with solutions containing ferritin, there is a strong correlation between the period of perfusion prior to fixation with osmium tetroxide and the number of vesicles labelled with ferritin, for perfusion periods of up to one

minute (fig. 1). This correlation between vesicular uptake of ferritin and time of exposure to tracer, suggests that: (I) prior to fixation, vesicles were present in the endothelial cell and that their contents were continually turning over or exchanging with the extracellular fluid; (II) if the composition of the fluid in the capillary lumen was changed then it took a minute or more to establish a new steady state composition for the average vesicular fluids; (III) we have demonstrated that the luminal vesicles were labelled more rapidly than the cytoplasmic vesicles, which were labelled more rapidly than the abluminal vesicles (fig. 1).

To account for this progressive labelling is difficult if vesicles are an artifact of chemical fixation. If all vesicles were formed as the fixative reacted with the proteins and lipids of the endothelial cells, causing the plasmalemmal membranes to invaginate, it is possible that some random labelling of the vesicles would occur. If the degree of labelling depended

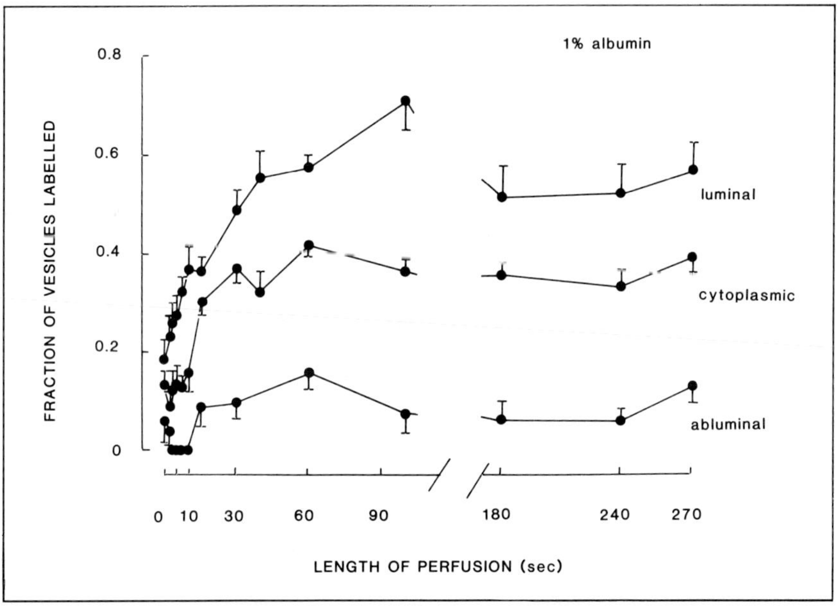

Fig. 1. The relationship between the fraction of luminal, cytoplasmic and abluminal vesicle populations labelled with molecules of ferritin (N_L/N_T) and the period of perfusion with a ferritin solution (6.7 g 100 ml^{-1}) containing 1 g 100 ml^{-1} bovine serum albumin, before fixation of the tissue with osmium tetroxide. Values are corrected for sectioning losses. Each point represents the mean and 95% confidence limits of a population of more than 100 vesicles taken from more than one experiment. Reprinted from [3].

upon the penetration of ferritin into the glycocalyx at the luminal surface [6], and it took a minute or more for the ferritin to come to equilibration with the interstices of the surface coat, then it could be possible for the uptake of ferritin into the luminal vesicles to correlate with time. On this hypothesis, however, there is no reason why the luminal vesicles should label more rapidly than cytoplasmic vesicles, or why any abluminal vesicles should be labelled.

We conclude that the progressive labelling of the vesicles with the length of exposure to ferritin before fixation, argues against the view that all vesicles are artifacts of chemical fixation.

(2) We have shown that the progressive labelling of vesicles with time prior to exposure to chemical fixatives, can be abolished by cooling the tissues to 4 °C (fig. 2). In cold tissues fixed with osmium tetroxide, the numbers of vesicles per μm^3 cell are similar to those found at 17 °C and the distribution of vesicles between the luminal, cytoplasmic and abluminal sites is also similar (table I). Thus, the same number of vesicles are present at 4 °C and 17 °C and they are distributed at the same sites within the cell. Yet, at 17 °C there is a progressive labelling with time up to 60 s,

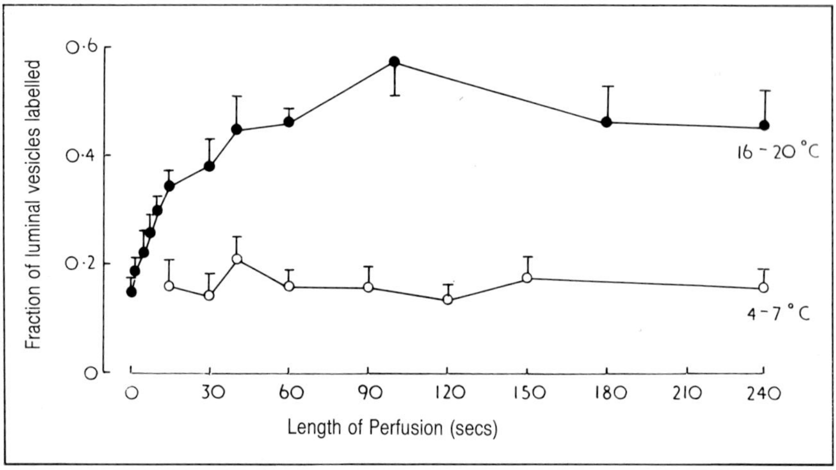

Fig. 2. The relationship between the fraction of the luminal vesicle populations labelled with ferritin molecules (N_L/N_T) and the period of exposure of the luminal cell surface to a ferritin solution (6.7 g 100 ml^{-1}) before fixation of the tissue with osmium tetroxide. Experiments were performed at 17–20 °C (closed circles) and at 4–7 °C (open circles). Values are corrected for sectioning losses. Each point represents the mean and 95% confidence limits of a population of more than 100 vesicles from more than one experiment. Reprinted from [4].

Table I. Diameter and distribution of vesicles in perfused frog capillaries

Fixation and temperature	Endothelial cell thickness (μm)	Frequency of vesicles L : C : A	Vesicle diameter (nm)	Luminal vesicles per μm^2 surface	Total vesicles per μm^3 cell
Osmium / 17 °C	0.26 ± 0.04	0.26:0.57:0.17	68.3 ± 1.3	23.7 ± 2.5	454 ± 46
Osmium / 4 °C	0.21 ± 0.02	0.25:0.53:0.21	64.0 ± 6.3	28.8 ± 3.0	629 ± 49
Glutaraldehyde/17 °C	0.13 ± 0.01	0.26:0.50:0.23	62.2 ± 1.6	33.7 ± 2.9	1277 ± 111

L = luminal; C = cytoplasmic; A = abluminal vesicles.
All values are mean ± 1 SEM

whereas at 4 °C there is no progressive labelling with time, merely the constant low level of labelling in all populations which is seen at zero time (i.e., when perfusion and fixation are simultaneous) at both 4 °C and 17 °C (figs. 1 and 3).

If the vesicles are formed by chemical fixation, it is difficult to see why they take up ferritin as they are formed at 17 °C but do not at 4 °C. A simpler explanation is that at 17 °C and 4 °C most of the vesicles seen in osmium-fixed tissue exist in vivo but the mechanism whereby they turn over their contents is inhibited at 4 °C.

(3) We have recently shown that if tissues are primarily fixed with glutaraldehyde rather than with osmium tetroxide, the numbers of vesicles per μm^3 endothelial cell increases 2–3 fold (table I). It has not yet been possible to demonstrate a time dependence of labelling using glutaraldehyde fixation, but the distribution of vesicles and the distribution of ferritin molecules in the vesicles appear similar to those seen in the steady state perfusions (> 1 min) fixed with osmium tetroxide. We are, however, unsure that such patterns of labelling following glutaraldehyde fixation are representative, as the time taken for glutaraldehyde to immobilize both the molecules of ferritin and the tissue membranes is known to be rather long and extremely variable.

Whereas we have recorded a small change in diameter of vesicles following glutaraldehyde fixation (about 10%) compared with that measured in osmium-fixed tissue (table I), the average thickness of the endothelium (Δx) fell to 0.14 to 0.12 μm with glutaraldehyde fixation compared with 0.21 to 0.26 μm with osmium tetroxide, i.e., $\Delta x_g = \frac{2}{3} \Delta x_{os}$ (assuming minimal values). If this represents shrinkage of the cell cytoplasm, one might expect that if the volume of the endothelium = V, then

$V_g = (2/3)^3 V_{os}$, where V_g and V_{os} are the apparent volumes after fixation with glutaraldehyde and osmium, respectively. If the numbers of vesicles per unit volume do not change, then this would represent an apparent increase in the total number of vesicles of 3 x, compared with our osmium fixed data and that of *Bundgaard and Frøkjær-Jensen* [1] using glutaraldehyde/formaldehyde fixation.

We conclude that the increase in the numbers of vesicles per unit volume of cell could merely indicate shrinkage of cytoplasm with glutaraldehyde or swelling of the cell cytoplasm with osmium tetroxide as the primary fixative.

(4) We have demonstrated that with osmium fixation, a small fraction of vesicles in all populations was labelled with ferritin molecules at zero time. This fraction of the cytoplasmic and abluminal populations did not increase with time over the first 10 s prior to fixation at 17 °C but did increase at later times. The same fraction of labelling was seen in all populations of vesicles at 4 °C and did not increase with time (fig. 3).

We suggested that these rapidly labelling vesicles could represent stable fusions of vesicles which opened directly on to the luminal surface [3, 4]. They could, however, be artifacts of chemical fixation – i. e., appli-

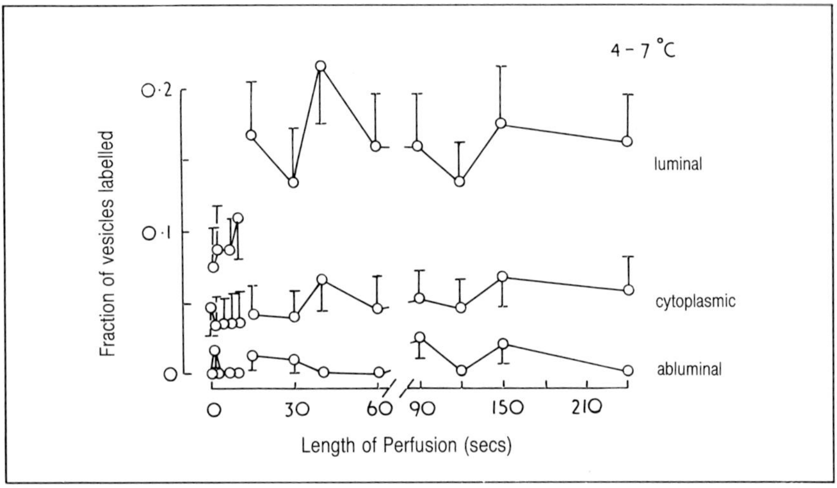

Fig. 3. The relationship between N_L/N_T for luminal, cytoplasmic and abluminal vesicle populations and the period of exposure of the luminal cell surface to a solution containing 6.7 g 100 ml^{-1} ferritin in tissue maintained at 4–7 °C and fixed with osmium tetroxide. Values estimated as in figures 1 and 2. Reprinted from [4].

cation of fixative causes new vesicles to form and fusions between vesicles at different sites in the cell to take place. A fraction of these new vesicles is then labelled.

If rapidly labelling vesicles are not artifacts, then a labelled caveola at the abluminal surface could be a channel [8]. The frequency of labelling of abluminal vesicles is about 1%. There are approximately 20 abluminal vesicles per μm^2 of luminal cell surface. Thus, there should be 1 channel per 5 μm^2 surface. This could make a major contribution to the hydrophilic pathway:

$$\text{let cell thickness be } \Delta x = 0.3\ \mu m,$$
$$\text{Radius (R) of vesicle neck} = 20\ nm,$$
$$\text{Then } \frac{Ap}{\Delta x} = \frac{\Pi\ (0.02\ \mu m)^2 / 5\ \mu m^2}{0.3\ \mu m}$$
$$= 0.00034\ \mu m^{-1}$$
$$= 8.4\ cm^{-1}$$

where A_p is the fraction of the membrane which is porous.

Since $A_p/\Delta x$ for frog capillaries $= 40\ cm^{-1}$, channels would account for 20% of the hydrophilic pathway.

Summary

We have used the individually perfused frog mesenteric capillary to investigate the possible contribution of endothelial cell vesicles to microvascular permeability. We have demonstrated that vesicles are unlikely to be an artifact of chemical fixation and that they have the ability to take up and transport tracer molecules across the endothelial cell. We have further shown that this transfer may be inhibited by reducing tissue temperature.

We have shown that the apparent size and the numbers of vesicles seen are partly dependent on the nature of the primary fixative used.

We have considered the possibility that the rapid labelling of vesicles across the cell at 17 °C and the labelling seen in the cold, might be an artifact of fixation. If it is not, and such labelling does represent the labelling of channels across the cell, formed by the fusion of vesicles, we have calculated that such channels would account for some 20% of the cell's hydraulic pathway and thus make a significant contribution to microvascular permeability.

Acknowledgment

The MRC are gratefully acknowledged for their financial support.

References

1 Bundgaard, M.; Frøkjær-Jensen, J.: Functional aspects of the ultrastructure of terminal blood vessels: A quantitative study on consecutive segments of the frog mesenteric microvasculature. Microvasc. Res. *23:* 1–30 (1982).
2 Clough, G.: The dependence of vesicular transport on various physiological parameters; in Messmer, Hammersen (eds.), Structure and function of endothelial cells, Prog. appl. Microcirc., vol. 1, pp. 35–50 (Karger, Basel 1983).
3 Clough, G.; Michel, C. C.: The role of vesicles in the transport of ferritin through frog endothelium. J. Physiol., Lond. *315:* 127–142 (1981).
4 Clough, G.; Michel, C. C.: The effects of temperature on ferritin transport by endothelial cell vesicles in the capillaries of the frog mesentery. Int. J. Microcirc.: Clin. Exp. *1:* 29–39 (1982).
5 Loudon, M. F.; Michel, C. C.; White, I. F.: The labelling of vesicles in frog endothelial cells with ferritin. J. Physiol., Lond. *296:* 97–112 (1979).
6 Michel, C. C.: The flow of water through the capillary wall; in Ussing, Bindslev, Lassen, Sten-Knudsen (eds.), Alfred Benzon Symposium 15, Water transport across epithelia, pp. 268–279 (Munksgaard, Copenhagen 1981).
7 Rippe, B.; Kamiya, A.; Folkow, B.: Is capillary micropinocytosis of any significance for the transcapillary transfer of plasma proteins. Acta physiol. scand. *100:* 258–260 (1977).
8 Simionescu, N.; Simionescu, M.: Hydrophilic pathways of capillary endothelium, a dynamic system; in Ussing, Bindslev, Lassen, Sten-Knudsen (eds.), Alfred Benzon Symposium 15, Water transport across epithelia, pp. 228–247 (Munksgaard, Copenhagen 1981).

Geraldine Clough, PhD, Department of Physiology and Biophysics, St. Mary's Hospital Medical School, London (England)

Prog. appl. Microcirc., vol. 9, pp. 59–66 (Karger, Basel 1985)

Vesicular Transport across Pulmonary Capillary Endothelium in the Fluorocarbon Exchange Transfused Rat

E. E. Schneeberger

Department of Pathology, Massachusetts General Hospital, Harvard Medical School, Boston, Mass., USA

Introduction

Experimentation with perfluorochemical-based blood substitutes began in 1965 with the extra-corporeal blood oxygenation experiments of *Howlett* et al. [7]. A year later *Clark and Gollan* reported that mice survived prolonged immersion in oxygenated liquid perfluorochemicals [1], and *Sloviter and Kamimoto* showed that perfusion with emulsified perfluorochemicals could sustain isolated rat brains for several hours [18]. By 1968 *Geyer* et al. [5] definitively demonstrated the capability of these compounds to sustain life following total blood replacement. These 'bloodless' rats were shown to behave in a normal manner and by 7 to 10 days the plasma protein concentration and hematocrit had returned to control levels [6]. The perfluorochemicals have the remarkable property of combining high O_2 and CO_2 solubility with extreme chemical and biological inertness [9]. They are commonly emulsified with Pluronic F-68 (Wyandotte Chemical Corp.) and hydroxyethyl starch is added as an oncotic agent. These emulsions, like blood, are non-Newtonian fluids which have a somewhat lower viscosity than blood and are, therefore, well suited to act as blood substitutes.

Advantage was taken of this 'bloodless' rat model to examine the effect of circulating proteins on vesicular transport across pulmonary capillary endothelium. From observations made in frog capillaries [4], it has long been known that circulating proteins interact with endothelial cells in such a way as to render the endothelium less permeable to water [12], small hydrophilic molecules [10] and macromolecules [2]. In the 'bloodless' rat model, it is possible, by meticulously controlling the osmolality of the perfluorochemical emulsion, to remove 99% of the animal's circulating protein without inducing pulmonary edema [14]. Morphometric studies were carried out in such animals to determine

(1) whether the perfluorochemical emulsion has any effect on the size and numerical density of endothelial vesicles and

(2) what effect the graded removal and replenishment of circulating proteins has on the vesicular transport of ferritin [13].

Material and Methods

All exchange transfusions were carried out on female Sprague-Dawley rats weighing 38–56 g. The exchange transfusions were carried out with Oxypherol-ET (Green Cross, Osaka, Japan), the composition of which was slightly modified as previously described [14]. The final osmolality ranged between 292–300 mOsm/kg and the pH was adjusted to 7.42 by gassing with 95% O_2 plus 5% CO_2.

The exchange transfusions were carried out as previously described [14]. In brief, following light ether anesthesia, the fluorocarbon emulsion was administered by a tail vein while blood was removed from the external jugular vein. A Harvard pump was modified to inject and withdraw samples simultaneously in order to maintain a constant blood volume. The animal breathed 90–100% O_2 to permit the use of relatively low concentrations of fluorocarbon. The exchange was carried out at a rate of 0.78 ml/min. At the end of an exchange, blood gas determinations were made and the concentration of circulating proteins determined by the method of *Lowry* et al. [11]. Wet to dry weight ratios were carried out on a group of 6 rats, exchange transfused with 1 ml/g BW of fluorocarbon emulsion.

Horse spleen ferritin, 2 times crystallized, was dialyzed, as previously described, to reduce its cadmium content [14]. At the end of an exchange, ferritin was administered intravenously over 1 min. The lungs were fixed by the intratracheal infusion of formaldehyde-glutaraldehyde fixative in 0.1 M cacodylate buffer 2–2.5 min after the start of the ferritin infusion. Following fixation in vitro in the same fixative for 4 h, the lungs were washed overnight in 0.15 M cacodylate buffer, pH 7.3.

The morphometric measurements, made on electron micrograph prints, were carried out by means of a Grafpen-40 (Science Accessories, Southport, CN) interfaced with a VAX11/780 computer. The computer was programmed to compute:

(1) Percent vesicles labeled with ferritin (% VL);

(2) number of ferritin particles per unit area of basement membrane (Fe/BM);

(3) mean vesicular diameter ($\overline{D}$);

(4) numerical density of endothelial vesicles per unit volume of endothelial cells (N_v); and

(5) endothelial fractional volume represented by vesicles (V_v).

Three types of experiments were carried out. In the first, to determine whether the perfluorochemicals had any effect on pulmonary endothelial N_v, $\overline{V}$ and V_v, animals were exchange transfused with 1 ml/g BW of fluorocarbon emulsion to reduce circulating proteins from 60 mg/ml to 0.4 mg/ml. The lungs were fixed and processed as previously described [14] and the morphometric measurements made on the thin and thick side of randomly selected pulmonary capillaries. These were compared with non-exchange transfused controls, the lungs of which were fixed the same way.

In the second set of experiments, circulating proteins were depleted in graded steps to result in circulating protein concentrations of 25, 10 or 4 mg/ml [13]. All rats were injected intravenously with 50 mg/100 g BW of native ferritin 2.5 min before sacrifice. Percent VL and Fe/BM were determined.

In the third group of experiments, circulating proteins were depleted to 1.1 mg/ml and the exchange transfusions were continued with fluorocarbon emulsions in which hydroxyethyl starch was partially or completely replaced by 15, 30, 45 or 60 mg/ml of lyophilized rat serum proteins. As in the second group of experiments, ferritin was injected intravenously 2.5 min before sacrifice and % VL and Fe/BM determined.

Results

Analysis of variance and covariance of the data shown in table I, indicated that there was no significant difference ($p > 0.1$) between exchange transfused and control rats in $\overline{D}$, N_v or V_v on either the thick or thin side of the capillaries. Vesicle $\overline{D}$, however, was larger on the thick than the thin side ($p < 0.0001$), while N_v was smaller on the thick than the thin side ($p < 0.0001$). As a result, V_v was similar on both sides of the capillaries.

Table I. Diameter, numerical density and fractional volume of vesicles in pulmonary capillaries of experimental and control rats

	Thick side of capillary			Thin side of capillary		
Group	$\overline{D}$	N_v	V_v	$\overline{D}$	N_v	V_v
Exchanged (5)	63.0 ±1.1	2.8 ±0.3	3.8 ±0.5	59.7 ±1.8	3.6 ±0.3	4.2 ±0.6
Control (5)	66.3 ±0.5	2.6 ±0.1	3.9 ±0.2	59.6 ±0.8	3.5 ±0.2	4.0 ±0.3

The numbers in parentheses indicate the number of rats in each group. The rats were exchange transfused with 1 ml/g BW of fluorocarbon emulsion. Values are means ± S. E. $\overline{D}$, mean vesicle diameter in nm, N_v, numerical density of vesicles per unit volume of endothelial cell × 10^{14} cm^{-3}; V_v, fractional volume of endothelial vesicles, × 10^{-2}.

In control rats, two and half minutes after the intravenous injection of ferritin, only 2.5% of endothelial vesicles contained ferritin on either the thin or the thick side of pulmonary capillaries. The labeled vesicles were either luminal or cytoplasmic in location and virtually none of the abluminal vesicles were labeled. Only a very small number of particles were observed in the basement membranes of either the thick or thin side of the capillary.

This was in marked contrast to the lungs from rats exchange transfused with 1 ml/g BW of fluorocarbon emulsion. In these animals, up to five times as many vesicles on both the thick and thin side of the capillaries were labeled (table II). As in control animals, most of the labeled vesicles were luminal and cytoplasmic in location. In addition, large numbers of ferritin particles were present in the basement membrane and their concentration was greater on the thick than the thin side of the capillary.

In the replenishment experiments, an analysis of the variance and covariance of the logarithmically transformed data showed that there was a significant inverse relationship between protein concentration and degree of vesicle labeling ($p < 0.001$), and that this effect was similar on both the thick and thin side of the capillary. A similar relationship between protein concentration and the amount of ferritin present in the basement membrane was observed. A protein concentration of 45 mg/ml

Table II. Effect of protein depletion and protein replenishment on percent vesicle labeling (% VL) and basement membrane labeling (Fe/BM) by Ferritin

Group	[Protein] (mg/ml)	VL (%)		Fe/BM Particles × 10^8 cm^{-2}	
		Thick	Thin	Thick	Thin
Protein Depletion	25	1.1 ± 0.1	0.8 ± 0.2	1.6 ± 0.2	2.0 ± 0.4
	10	1.4 ± 0.5	0.7 ± 0.2	2.3 ± 0.3	2.5 ± 1.0
	4	1.2 ± 0.3	1.2 ± 0.4	10.6 ± 2.8	9.8 ± 3.1
	0.5	5.1 ± 1.0	4.4 ± 1.0	15.0 ± 3.6	13.1 ± 2.8
Protein Replenishment	15	2.9 ± 0.4	2.3 ± 0.2	14.9 ± 3.8	14.9 ± 4.7
	30	2.6 ± 0.5	2.3 ± 0.5	4.8 ± 0.8	4.7 ± 1.6
	60	1.1 ± 0.2	0.8 ± 0.2	1.1 ± 0.4	1.5 ± 0.6

The data are means ± S.E. of triplicate experiments normalized to control values. % VL, percent vesicles labeled, Fe/BM, number of ferritin particles × 10^8 per unit area of basement membrane.

was sufficient to return the degree of basement membrane labeling by ferritin on the thin side to control levels. On the thick side, however, 60 mg/ml of protein was necessary to achieve control values. At the latter concentration, the degree of vesicle and basement membrane labeling was indistinguishable from that of controls (table II).

In contrast to the repletion phase, depletion of protein to 4 mg/ml had no effect on % VL. Furthermore, during depletion, a protein concentration as low as 25 mg/ml was sufficient to maintain Fe/BM at control levels (table II). These results suggest an hysteresis effect: during repletion 2.5 times more protein was necessary to maintain normal macromolecular permeability to ferritin than during depletion.

Discussion

The fluorocarbon exchange transfused rat provides a unique model in which to study vesicular transport functions in the intact animal. In the studies reviewed here, it was found that extensive exchange transfusions carried out with perfluorochemical emulsions had no effect on the distribution, size or numerical density of endothelial vesicles in pulmonary capillaries. On the other hand, the virtually complete removal of circulating proteins resulted in a 5 and 10-fold increase, respectively, in vesicular and basement membrane labeling by ferritin. This phenomenon was completely reversible, but required 60 mg/ml of lyophilized rat serum protein in order to achieve control levels. In contrast, during the graded depletion of circulating proteins, as little as 25 mg/ml of circulating proteins was sufficient to maintain normal endothelial permeability to ferritin. An analogous hysteresis effect for graded protein concentration on the hydraulic conductivity of frog capillaries has been observed: after Ringer's perfusion, a 10-fold higher concentration of protein was necessary to reduce the hydraulic conductivity to control levels [8].

The effect of circulating proteins on the permeability properties of the capillary wall has been attributed to the direct interaction of proteins with the glycocalyx on the surface of endothelial cells. In their fiber matrix model, *Curry and Michel* [3] visualized the glycocalyx as a meshwork of glycoprotein fibers, 0.6 nm in radius, and occupying less than 8% of the network volume. The trapping of protein in the network would effectively tighten the mesh and make the underlying luminal vesicles less accessible to other water-soluble molecules.

This phenomenon has been examined directly in the fluorocarbon exchange transfused rat by immunoperoxidase techniques [15]. In brief, it was shown that after depleting circulating proteins to 0.4 mg/ml, no immunocytochemically demonstrable albumin or immunoglobulin G was present in the alveolar wall. Three and a half minutes after the intravenous administration of 60 mg of lyophilized rat serum protein, a thin layer of reaction product was present in, and largely confined to, the endothelial glycocalyx. A few luminal vesicles contained reaction product as well, but, more importantly, the permeability of the vessels to native ferritin was indistinguishable from that of controls. These observations support the *Curry and Michel* fiber matrix model [3], and suggest that the presence of adsorbed proteins on the surface of the endothelium sterically hinders the access of ferritin to the luminal vesicles.

It has been suggested (Karnovsky, personal communication), that the interpretation of morphometric data of endothelial vesicles in aldehyde fixed tissue may be more complex than previously assumed, since fewer vesicles are observed when unfixed endothelium is processed by rapid freezing techniques. On the other hand, it remains to be established which of the two techniques preserves tissue most closely to the in vivo state. In a recent study, for example, of the endothelial vesicular system in fetal lamb lungs following aldehyde fixation, there was a 10-fold increase in the numerical density of endothelial cell vesicles from the glandular to the end of the alveolar stage of fetal development [16]. An identical fixation protocol was used at all stages of lung development. Interestingly, the numerical density of endothelial coated vesicles remained constant during this time span. Further studies are required to establish what the structure-function relationships of endothelial vesicles in the living state are.

Summary

The present studies clearly show that the fluorocarbon exchange transfused rat provides a versatile model in which to study the dynamics and mechanisms of vesicular transport in the intact animal. By using this model and native ferritin as a tracer molecule, it has been shown that there is a significant inverse relationship between circulating protein concentration and the relative number of vesicles labeled by ferritin and the number of ferritin particles in the basement membrane. An hysteresis effect was observed: in repletion experiments almost 2.5 times more protein was required to maintain capillary permeability at normal levels than during depletion experiments.

Acknowledgment

This study was supported by NIH Grant HL25822. The expert typing skills of Mr. *William Nelson* are gratefully acknowledged.

References

1 Clark, L. C.; Gollan, F.: Survival of mammals breathing organic liquids equilibrated with oxygen at atmospheric pressure. Science *152:* 1755–1756 (1966).
2 Clough, G.; Michel, C. C.: The role of vesicles in the transport of ferritin through frog endothelium. J. Physiol., Lond. *315:* 127–142 (1981).
3 Curry, F. E.; Michel, C. C.: A fiber matrix model of capillary permeability. Microvasc. Res. *20:* 96–99 (1980).
4 Drinker, C. K.: The permeability and diameter of the capillaries in the web of the brown frog *(Rana temporaria)* when perfused with solutions containing pituitary extract and horse serum. J. Physiol., Lond. *63:* 249–269 (1927).
5 Geyer, R. P.; Monroe, R. G.; Taylor, K.: Survival of rats having red cells totally replaced with emulsified fluorocarbon. Fed. Proc. *27:* 384 (1968).
6 Geyer, R. P.: 'Bloodless' rats through the use of artificial blood substitutes. Fed. Proc. *34:* 1499–1505 (1975).
7 Howlett, S.; Dundas, D.; Sabiston, D. C.: Fluid fluorocarbon as oxygenator in experimental extracorporeal circulation. Archs. Surg. *91:* 643–645 (1965).
8 Huxley, V. H.; Curry, F. E.: Graded effect of albumin concentration on the hydraulic conductivity of frog capillaries. Microvasc. Res. *23:* 259 (1982).
9 LeBlanc, M.; Riess, J. G.: Artificial blood substitutes based on perfluorochemicals; in Banks (ed.), Preparation, properties and industrial applications of organofluorine compounds, pp. 83–138 (John Wiley & Sons, New York 1982).
10 Levick, J. R.; Michel, C. C.: The effect of bovine albumin on the permeability of frog mesenteric capillaries Q. Jl exp. Physiol. *58:* 87–97 (1973).
11 Lowry, O. H.; Rosebrough, N. J.; Farr, A.; Randall, R. J.: Protein measurement with the folin phenol reagent. J. biol. Chem. *193:* 265–275 (1951).
12 Mason, J. C.; Curry, F. E.; Michel, C. C.: The effect of proteins upon the filtration coefficient of individually perfused frog mesenteric capillaries. Microvasc. Res. *13:* 185–202 (1977).
13 Schneeberger, E. E.; Hamelin, M.; Neary, B. A.; McCormack, J. M.: Graded effect of circulating protein concentration on ferritin transport across pulmonary endothelium. Microvasc. Res. *25:* 255 (1983).
14 Schneeberger, E. E.; Neary, B. A.: The bloodless rat: a new model for macromolecular transport studies across lung endothelium. Am. J. Physiol. *242:* H890–H899 (1982).
15 Schneeberger, E. E.; Hamelin, M.: Interaction of plasma proteins with lung endothelial glycocalyx: its effect on endothelial permeability. Am. J. Physiol. *247:* H206–H217 (1984).
16 Schneeberger, E. E.: Plasmalemmal vesicles in pulmonary capillary endothelium of developing fetal lamb lungs. Microvasc. Res. *25:* 40–55 (1983).

17 Schneeberger, E. E.: The use of PFC exchange transfused rats in studies of lung microvascular permeability; in Bolin, Geyer, Nemo (eds.), Advances in blood substitute research, pp. 249–256 (Liss, New York 1983).
18 Sloviter, H. A.; Kamimoto, T.: Erythrocyte substitute for perfusion of brain. Nature, Lond. *216:* 458–460 (1967).

Eveline E. Schneeberger, MD, Department of Pathology, Massachusetts General Hospital, Harvard Medical School, Boston, MA 02114 (USA)

Prog. appl. Microcirc., vol. 9, pp. 67–79 (Karger, Basel 1985)

Morphometric Studies of Endothelial Vesicles of Alveolar Vessels in Edematous Lungs

D. O. DeFouw

Department of Anatomy, New Jersey Medical School, Newark, N. J., USA

Introduction

The principal focus of the studies described in this report is directed toward morphologic changes in capillary endothelia after hemodynamic pulmonary edema formation. Increased filtration rates from alveolar microvessels during the onset of hemodynamic edema are attributed primarily, but not solely, to alterations of microvascular hydrostatic and/or oncotic pressures [16]. Based on Starling's hypothesis, changes in microvessel hydrostatic or colloid osmotic pressures represent an accentuation of the normal process of fluid exchange across pulmonary microvessel endothelia [13] with consequent fluid accumulation within interstitial spaces surrounding the alveolar microvessels, extra-alveolar vessels and airways [4, 21].

Ultrastructural morphometric analyses of alveolar microvessels in edematous lungs are presented here with particular emphasis on endothelial plasmalemmal vesicles. Comparisons of various models of acute hemodynamic edema formation in isolated dog lungs, and dog lungs in vivo, serve to address the temporal relation of extravascular fluid accumulation and observed alterations in the endothelial vesicle populations. Since these ultrastructural studies are based upon established stereologic techniques [25], the importance of this powerful morphological research procedure is exemplified.

Material and Methods

Isolated perfused lungs

Detailed descriptions of the isolated perfused lung preparations were presented previously [6, 7]. Briefly, isolated lungs, maintained with positive pressure ventilation, were perfused at a constant rate with cell-free perfusate, which consisted of 6% dextran in a modified Ringer's solution at 37 °C. Hydrostatic edema was produced in a series of isolated lungs by progressively elevating venous out-flow pressures over periods of 30–45 min [6]. Oncotic edema was produced in another experimental series by incremental replacement of perfusate with equal volumes of normal saline over periods of 45–60 min [7]. The lungs in both series were subsequently fixed by tracheal instillation of 2% glutaraldehyde in 0.15 M bicarbonate buffer at 20 cm H_2O pressure. For comparative purposes, another hydrostatic edema series was completed by employing vascular-perfusion fixation rather than tracheal instillation of fixative [8]. A series of isolated lung preparations, perfused at 15 °C, was also evaluated after hydrostatic edema formation [3]. The final series of isolated lung preparations served to compare alveolar microvessels after sequential induction of moderate and severe hydrostatic edema at 37 °C [11].

In vivo lungs

Descriptions of the circulatory overload and plasmapheresis procedures were presented elsewhere [9]. Hydrostatic edema was produced by circulatory overload during which an infusion solution of 4% bovine serum albumin, containing red blood cells, was pumped into the cannulated femoral vein. Oncotic edema was produced by plasmapheresis during which blood was withdrawn from the femoral artery, mixed with saline or dextran, and centrifuged to obtain the erythrocytes. The cells were then combined with saline and reinfused into the femoral vein. After completion of the overload or plasmapheresis procedures, the lungs were fixed via tracheal instillation of buffered glutaraldehyde.

Ultrastructural morphometry

24 tissue blocks were taken from each of the fixed lungs according to a stratified sampling procedure [25]. The tissue blocks were postfixed in 1% osmium tetroxide in 0.15 M bicarbonate buffer, dehydrated in graded ethanols and propylene oxide, and embedded in Epon. 10 blocks were chosen randomly from the primary sample of 24 blocks for ultramicrotomy. Ultrathin sections from each of the 10 blocks were obtained at a thickness of 75 nm, as judged by their silver-gold interference color. A single thin section from each block was used to generate six electron micrographs of the alveolar septa at an initial magnification of × 960 and another six micrographs of the capillary endothelia at × 12,180 initial magnification. Thus, a total of 120 micrographs was obtained from each of the experimental lungs.

The segment of alveolar septa presented in each micrograph was either evaluated in toto or was demarcated into its thin and thick sides, which are structurally distinct on the two dimensional micrographs (fig. 1). The capillary endothelial and alveolar epithelial basal laminae are separated by interstitial cells and fibers on the thick sides of the septa. Apparent

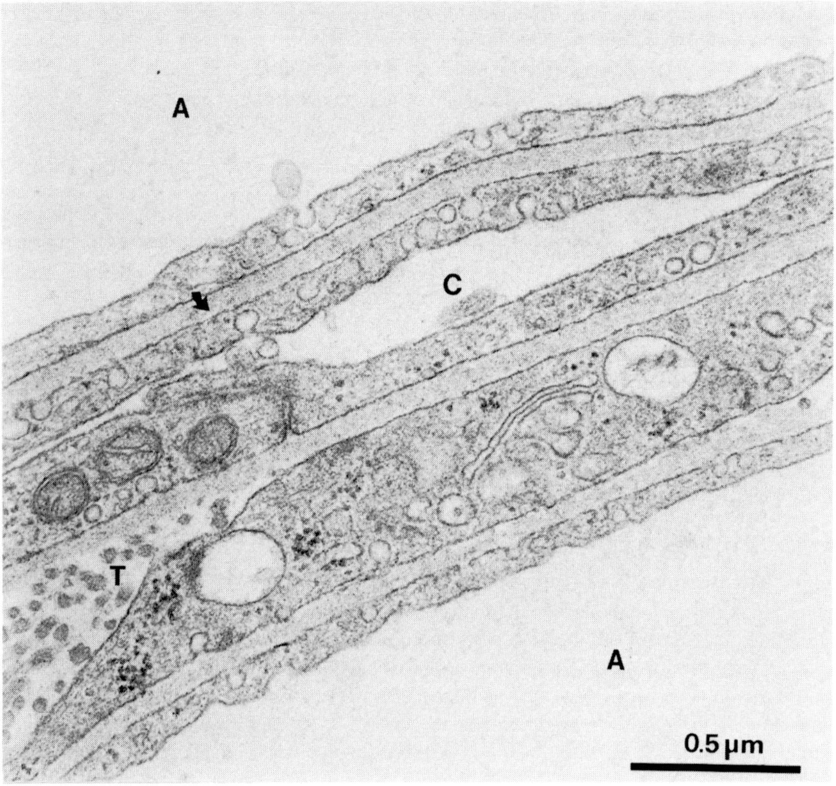

Fig. 1. A segment from an alveolar septum of a nonedematous isolated perfused dog lung is illustrated. The thin side of the septum (small arrow) is comprised of the apparently fused basal laminae from the type I epithelium, which lines the alveoli (A), and the endothelium of the alveolar capillary (C). The thick side of the septum (T) is characterized by separation of the respective basal laminae by a segment of an interstitial cell and scattered collagen fibrils. Approximate magnification 45,000×.

fusion of the respective basal laminae into a single lamina is observed on the thin sides. The morphometric observations were categorized as from the thick sides of the septa, the thin sides of the septa, or from the total septa.

A stereologic grid, composed of 84 lines and 168 points in the form of a transparent overlay, was used to obtain morphometric data from each micrograph. Line intercepts, point counts, and plasmalemmal vesicle enumerations were recorded to obtain estimates of the morphometric parameters. Mean arithmetic thicknesses (expressed as volume to surface ratios) of the microvessel endothelia or the endothelial cytoplasmic compartments were calculated from the micrographs as:

$$t = \frac{d \cdot Pc}{4 \cdot Ic}$$

where d represents the calibrated length of a single line; Pc is the number of points superimposed on either the entire endothelium or the endothelial cytoplasmic profiles; Ic is the number of line intersections with the endothelial luminal surface profiles [23].

Endothelial vesicle volume densities were determined on the micrographs at × 12,180 initial magnification according to:

$$Vv = \frac{Pv}{Pv+Pc}$$

where Pv is the number of points superimposed on the endothelial vesicle profiles and Pc is the number of points on the endothelial cytoplasm [25]. The vesicle numerical densities within the endothelial cytoplasmic compartments were calculated as:

$$Nv = \frac{Na}{\overline{D}+T-2h}$$

where Na is the number of profiles counted per unit area of endothelial cytoplasm; $\overline{D}$ represents equatorial diameters of the vesicles; T is thickness of the ultrathin sections; h represents the depth by which a vesicle must penetrate the section before it is detected. Vesicle diameters were measured at their most circular part and the vesicles were assumed to be spherical in shape. Approximately 200–300 vesicles were measured in the endothelial cytoplasm on both the thin and thick sides of the alveolar septa. The mean profile diameter method [14] was used to estimate vesicle diameters. The frequency distribution graphs constructed for this method contained radii of the smallest visible vesicle profiles identifiable in the tissue sections. These values were used to determine h [24].

The extent of endothelial attenuation was determined from the micrographs at × 12,180 original magnification. Relative proportions of total endothelial surface occupied by extremely thin cytoplasmic attenuations (approximately 30–40 nm thick), and by cytoplasmic segments with thicknesses greater than 40 nm, were differentiated.

Mean values for the morphometric parameters were determined for each experimental group and differences between means were tested for significance by an unpaired t-test or a one way analysis of variance. Statistical significance was accepted at $p<0.05$.

Results

Since alterations in the relations between pulmonary microvascular hydrostatic and oncotic pressures are the principal determinants of hemodynamic edema formation [13, 16], increases in perfusion pressure or decreases in perfusate oncotic pressure in isolated perfused lungs served as the initial experimental model [6–8]. In each of these studies, the lungs were sampled after extensive extravascular fluid accumulation and alveolar flooding. The morphometric data in table I indicate an absence of cellular edema, even though the interstitial compartment of the alveolar septa contained extensive fluid accumulation (fig. 2). Vesicle volume densities in the capillary endothelia were nearly doubled after the production of either type of hydrodynamic edema. Further, the route of

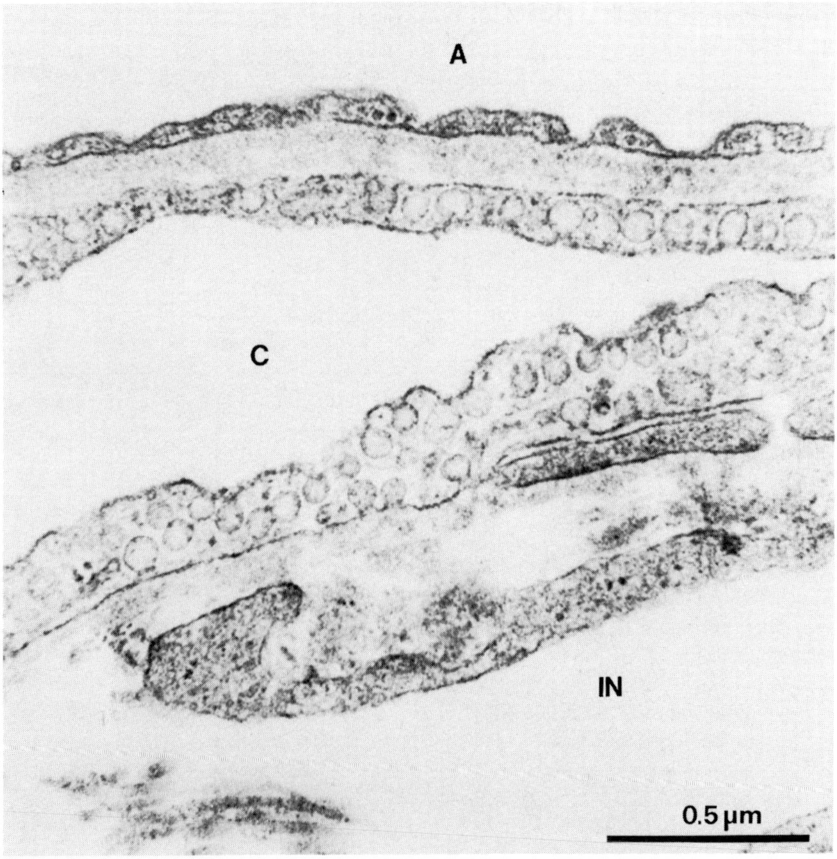

Fig. 2. This segment of an alveolar septum from an edematous isolated dog lung preparation depicts the accumulation of fluid on the thick side of the septum (IN). The thin side is not noticeably altered but the capillary (C) endothelium presents extensive vesiculation on both the thin and thick sides of the septum. Approximate magnification 54,000 ×.

fixative administration (instillation or perfusion) did not influence the vesicular response to the edematous conditions.

Since alveolar flooding represents the final stage of edema formation [21], additional isolated perfused lung preparations were evaluated prior to the alveolar flooding stage. Morphometric evaluations of these preparations were made after induction of extravascular fluid accumulation, which was restricted to the interstitial spaces surrounding alveolar and extra-alveolar pulmonary vessels and the large airways [11]. The interpretation that alveolar microvessel plasmalemmal vesicles increased in volume density after septal interstitial edema, but prior to alveolar flooding, is consistent with the data presented in table II.

The data in tables I and II also provide evidence for the suggestion that vesicle volume densities increased in the edematous lungs as a result of increases in vesicle numbers rather than increases in vesicle sizes. The estimates of vesicle numerical densities, presented in table III, provide

Table I. Alveolar capillary endothelia in isolated perfused dog lungs after acute, severe hydrostatic or oncotic edema formation*

	Control	Edema	
		Hydrostatic	Oncotic
Endothelial cell thickness (μm)			
Instillation fixation	0.34 ± 0.01	0.37 ± 0.01	0.33 ± 0.01
Vascular fixation	0.30 ± 0.02	0.28 ± 0.05	
Vesicle volume density			
Instillation fixation	26.0 ± 1.4	46.0 ± 3.4**	42.0 ± 5.2*
Vascular fixation	21.7 ± 2.4	30.61 ± 0.75**	
Vesicle diameter (nm)			
Instillation fixation	63.5 ± 1.1	66.5 ± 1.8	67.6 ± 2.5
Vascular fixation	60.8 ± 2.3	57.9 ± 3.9	

* Data from [6, 7, 8]
** $p < 0.025$

Table II. Alveolar capillary endothelia in isolated perfused lungs after production of acute, moderate and severe hydrostatic edema*

	Control	Edema	
		Moderate	Severe
Endothelial cell thickness (μm)	0.25 ± 0.06	0.24 ± 0.03	0.26 ± 0.07
Vesicle volume density (% cytoplasm)	8.9 ± 1.4	16.8 ± 2.5**	15.3 ± 2.9**
Vesicle diameter (nm)	67.7 ± 5.5	71.4 ± 1.0	73.0 ± 2.6

* Data from [11]
** $p < 0.05$

further support to this interpretation. An important ultrastructural distinction of capillary endothelia on the thin and thick sides of the alveolar septa is also presented in table III. In nonedematous and edematous lungs the extent of endothelial attenuation was markedly greater on the thin sides of the septa and thus, overall cytoplasmic thickness was less on the thin sides. Further, endothelial vesicle numerical densities were substantially greater on the thin sides of the septa. Whether these ultrastructural variations are associated with functional differences between endothelia on the thin and thick sides of the septa remains uncertain. However, it should be emphasized that greater vesicle numerical densities on the thin sides cannot be accounted for on the basis of vesicle displacement from the portion of cytoplasm that had become thinned out (attenuated), because calculation of vesicle densities takes into account the total cytoplasmic volume.

Are increased numbers of endothelial vesicles associated with increased outward filtration from the pulmonary microcirculation, thus contributing to edema formation? This question was initially tested by using both the isolated perfused dog lung preparations [3], and dog lungs in vivo [9]. After development of increased outward filtration with consequent interstitial edema and alveolar flooding in isolated lungs, perfused at 15 °C, endothelial vesicle volume densities and mean vesicle diameters

Table III. Comparative morphometric data from capillary endothelia on the thin and thick sides of the alveolar septa after acute, severe hydrostatic edema formation in isolated dog lungs*

	Thin Side		Thick Side	
	Control	Edema	Control	Edema
Cytoplasmic thickness (μm)	0.10 ± 0.01	0.11 ± 0.02	0.16 ± 0.04**	0.15 ± 0.03**
Percent cellular attenuation	16 ± 3	25 ± 11	< 1**	2 ± 1**
Vesicle numerical density (number/μm³ cytoplasm)	358 ± 46	653 ± 86***	258 ± 36**	485 ± 35***
Vesicle diameter (nm)	60 ± 3	60 ± 2	60 ± 2	60 ± 4

* Data from [10]

** Significant differences between controls on the thin and thick sides or between edematous samples on the thin and thick sides

*** Significant differences between the control and edematous samples on the respective sides of the septa remained unchanged (table IV). These results support the concept that normal lipid fluidity in the lipid bilayer of the endothelial plasmalemma is a major factor in plasmalemmal vesicle formation. Further, the occurrence of edema without increased endothelial vesiculation does not provide support for the concept that capillary endothelial vesicles play a major, early role in the development of pulmonary edema. Additional experimental evidence, which served to negate a contribution of increased endothelial vesiculation to edema formation, was provided by the morphometric data presented in table V. After increased outward filtration from the pulmonary microcirculation had been induced by circulatory overload or plasmapheresis in dog lungs in vivo, extravascular fluid accumulation was found in the extraalveolar connective tissue spaces while alveolar septal edema was not observed. Further, capillary endothelial vesicle diameters and hence, vesicle volume densities were markedly reduced. The stimulus for this reduction in vesicle sizes remains uncertain. However, the results of this study support the tentative hypothesis that increased alveolar septal interstitial pressures play a role in initiating endothelial vesicle formation

Table IV. Capillary endothelial vesicles after acute, severe edema formation in isolated dog lungs, perfused at 15 °C*

	Control	Edema
Vesicles		
Volume density	20.7 ± 3.4	22.1 ± 3.3
Mean diameter (nm)	63.0 ± 2.0	64.0 ± 2.0

* Data from [3]

Table V. Capillary endothelia in dog lungs in vivo after circulatory overload and plasmapheresis*

	Normal	Overload	Plasmapheresis
Endothelial cell thickness (μm)	0.27 ± 0.05	0.23 ± 0.03	0.25 ± 0.01
Vesicle volume density	26.4 ± 2.2	16.8 ± 0.9**	17.4 ± 1.5**
Vesicle diameter (nm)	70.7 ± 2.1	59.7 ± 1.5**	60.7 ± 0.6**

* Data from [9]
** $p < 0.05$

[2]. That is, if the increased outward filtration to be expected from the increased hydrostatic or decreased oncotic pressures was accommodated by increased flow rates in the intact lymph vessels, fluid accumulation in the alveolar septal interstitium, and presumed increases in septal interstitial pressures, would be diminished. Thus, if postulated increases in interstitial pressures were less than in the previously described isolated perfused lung preparations, failure to detect an increase in capillary endothelial vesicle volume densities is consistent with this hypothesis.

Discussion

The stereologic properties of vesicle volume densities and endothelial cell volume to surface ratios can be estimated from the two-dimensional electron micrographs without any restricting geometric assumptions [12]. Estimates of vesicle size distributions, on the other hand, require assumptions that vesicles are spherical in shape and that their diameters are normally distributed [15]. In addition, the mean profile diameter method [14] used in these studies relies on a somewhat empiric correction for missed vesicle profiles [5]. Corrections for truncation and overprojection of vesicle profiles are included in the stereologic formula for calculating vesicle numerical densities [25]; however, the corrections are based upon the estimates of mean vesicle profile diameters and of thicknesses of the ultrathin tissue sections. Thus, vesicle numerical densities presented in this report represent a rough estimation of vesicle number; however, comparisons between this morphometric parameter in the nonedematous and edematous lungs were not compromised and served to identify significant differences after edema formation.

The influence of overprojection (Holmes effect) on estimates of vesicle volume densities is illustrated by the approximate 3-fold discrepancy in vesicle volume densities presented in tables I and IV compared to those listed in table II for the isolated lung preparations. The data in table II was obtained by including a correction factor for tissue section thickness and, in this way, the overestimation of vesicle densities which results when section thickness is greater than vesicle diameters was compensated. Application of a correction factor for section thickness [24] to the data presented in tables I and IV yields respective endothelial vesicle volume densities of approximately 10 and 15% in the nonedematous and edematous lungs. Therefore, the results from each of the isolated lung preparations are reasonably consistent when appropriate corrections for tissue section thickness are incorporated.

Results from the studies described here provide the basis for the suggestion that endothelial vesicles are not primarily associated with edema formation. Thus, the increase in number of vesicles after development of hemodynamic edema, which has been confirmed by others [18], is viewed as a secondary event, perhaps a defense mechanism, in response to increased tissue pressure [2]. The defense mechanism would provide retrograde transport of water and other molecules, which had access to the vesicles, from the alveolar septal interstitium to the vascular compartment. In this way, a mechanism to limit interstitial accumulation of water and solutes which had entered the interstitium by any accessible route (e.g., endothelial junctions), might be provided by the vesicular system. Alternatively, the expanded vesicular population might signify an initial pathologic response of the capillary endothelial cells, with subsequent coalescence of the more closely packed vesicles eventually leading to cytoplasmic vacuole formation and ultimately to disruption of the endothelial lining layer.

The possible role of endothelial vesicles in water and solute exchange has been the subject of several recent reviews [e.g., 19, 20, 22]. It is generally considered that vesicles present a means of exchange for water, small solutes, and macromolecules between the vascular and interstitial compartments; however, mechanisms which regulate net directional exchange remain uncertain. Whether vesicles and their presumably derivative structures, e.g., branching invaginations from the plasmalemma [1], are static and effectively decrease cellular thickness, provide transcellular channels, or participate in a shuttle mechanism, remain provoking questions for a number of laboratories.

The hypothesis that increased septal interstitial pressures could contribute to increased capillary endothelial vesiculation should also be extended to include the contribution of interstitial pressure to endothelial cell attenuation [10]. Interestingly, the endothelia on the thin sides of the septa, relative to the thick sides, contain greater numbers of vesicles and display a greater extent of cellular attenuation in both the nonedematous and edematous lungs. If it is assumed, though not verified, that the fused basal laminae on the septal thin sides are less compliant than the interstitium on the thick sides (extracellular septal edema is restricted to the thick sides), the effects of perfusion pressures in the nonedematous lungs, coupled with alveolar flooding in the edematous lungs, could result in application of greater pressures to the endothelia on the thin sides. Further, the report that endothelial cell junctions are most numerous on the septal thick sides [17], in conjunction with the morphometric evidence that vesicles are most numerous on the thin sides, identifies the need for additional investigation of the contribution of vesicles to endothelial cell activity in normal and edematous lungs.

Summary

Pulmonary capillary endothelial vesicle numerical densities were approximately doubled in isolated perfused lungs after development of septal edema and alveolar flooding. The formation of similarly edematous conditions in isolated lungs perfused at 15 °C failed to increase the number of endothelial vesicles. Further, extravascular fluid accumulation, restricted to the extra-alveolar connective tissue spaces, in dog lungs in vivo was not accompanied by increased capillary endothelial vesiculation. The results of these quantitative morphologic studies are consistent with the interpretation that first, increased capillary endothelial vesiculation requires normal fluidity of the plasmalemmal lipid bilayer and second, it is not associated with increased rates of outward filtration from the alveolar microvascular beds in the absence of septal edema. A tentative hypothesis has evolved to the effect that increased septal interstitial pressures serve as a stimulus to endothelial vesicle formation which is then viewed as a defense mechanism against extensive interstitial fluid accumulation by providing a retrograde pathway for excess filtrate into the blood. The expanded vesicle population, on the other hand, could signify a cellular pathologic response to the edematous conditions.

Acknowledgment

The author thanks Dr. *F. P. Chinard* for his suggestions and Dr. *P. Chowdhury*, Mrs. *Perlita Hill*, Miss *Gail Smith*, Mrs. *Gertrude Anderson*, and the late Mr. *Gary Schroller* for their technical assistance. This work was supported by a Grant-in-Aid from The American Heart Association with funds contributed in part by the New Jersey Affiliate and the Bergen-Passaic and Ocean County Chapters and by Public Health Service Grant HL 19 571.

References

1 Bundgaard, M.; Frøkjær-Jensen, J.; Crone, C.: Endothelial plasmalemmal vesicles as elements in a system of branching invaginations from the cell surface. Proc. natn. Acad. Sci. USA *76:* 6439–6442 (1979).

2 Chinard, F. P.: Pulmonary endothelial and epithelial vesiculation as a response to increased blood-to-tissue filtration. Physiologist *23:* 62–66 (1980).

3 Chinard, F. P.; DeFouw, D. O.: Ultrastructural changes of the air-blood barrier after spontaneous development of edema in isolated dog lungs perfused at 15 °C. Microvasc. Res. *21:* 48–56 (1981).
4 Cottrell, T. S.; Levine, O. R.; Senior, R. M; Wiener, J.; Spiro, D.; Fishman, A. P.: Electron microscopic alterations at the alveolar level in pulmonary edema. Circulation Res. *21:* 783–797 (1967).
5 Cruz-Orive, L. M.: Distribution-free estimation of sphere size distributions from slabs showing overprojection and truncation, with a review of previous methods. J. Microscopy, Oxford *131:* 265–290 (1983).
6 DeFouw, D. O.; Berendsen, P. B.: Morphological changes in isolated perfused dog lungs after acute hydrostatic edema. Circulation Res. *43:* 72–82 (1978).
7 DeFouw, D. O.; Berendsen, P. B.: A morphometric analysis of isolated perfused dog lungs after acute oncotic edema. Microvasc. Res. *17:* 90–103 (1979).
8 DeFouw, D. O.: Morphologic study of the alveolar septa in normal and edematous isolated dog lungs fixed by vascular perfusion. Lab. Invest. *42:* 413–419 (1980).
9 DeFouw, D. O.; Cua, W. O.; Chinard, F. P.: Morphometric and physiological studies of alveolar microvessels in dog lungs in vivo after sustained increases in pulmonary microvascular pressures and after sustained decreases in plasma oncotic pressures. Microvasc. Res. *25:* 56–67 (1983).
10 DeFouw, D. O.; Chinard, F. P.: Variations in cellular attenuation and vesicle numerical densities in capillary endothelium and type I epithelium of isolated perfused dog lungs after acute severe edema formation. Microvasc. Res. *26:* 15–26 (1983).
11 DeFouw, D. O.; Ritter, A. B.; Chinard, F. P.: Alveolar vessels in isolated perfused dog lungs: structural and functional studies after production of moderate and severe hydrodynamic edema. Exp. Lung Res. *8:* 67 (1985).
12 DeHoff, R. T.: Quantitative serial sectioning analysis: preview. J. Microscopy, Oxford *131:* 259–263 (1983).
13 Garr, K. A.; Taylor, A. E.; Owens, L. J.; Guyton, A. C.: Effects of capillary pressure and plasma protein on development of pulmonary edema. Am. J. Physiol. *213:* 79–82 (1967).
14 Giger, H.; Riedwyl, H.: Bestimmung der Größenverteilung von Kugeln aus Schnittkreisradien. Biometr. Z. *12:* 156–174 (1970).
15 Greeley, D. A.; Crapo, J. D.: Practical approach to the estimation of overall mean caliper diameter of a population of spheres and its application to data where small profiles are missed. J. Microscopy, Oxford *114:* 261–269 (1978).
16 Guyton, A. C.; Lindsey, A. W.: Effect of elevated left atrial pressures and decreased protein concentration on the development of pulmonary edema. Circulation Res. *7:* 649–657 (1959).
17 Hurley, J. V.: Current views on the mechanisms of pulmonary edema. J. Pathol. *125:* 59–79 (1978).
18 Mazzone, R. W.; Kornblau, S. M.: Influence of vascular and transpulmonary pressures on endothelial vesicles in nonedematous and edematous lungs. Microvasc. Res. *25:* 343–357 (1983).
19 Renkin, E. M.: Multiple pathways of capillary permeability. Circulation Res. *41:* 735–743 (1977).
20 Simionescu, N.: Hydrophilic pathways of capillary endothelium, a dynamic system; in

Ussing, Bindslev, Lassen, Sten-Knudsen (eds.), Alfred Benzon Symposium 15, Water transport across epithelia, pp. 228–247 (Munksgaard, Copenhagen 1981).
21 Staub, N. C.; Nagano, H.; Pearce, M. L.: Pulmonary edema in dogs, especially the sequence of fluid accumulation in lungs. J. appl. Physiol. *22:* 227–240 (1967).
22 Wagner, R. C.; Casley Smith, J. R.: Review: endothelial vesicles. Microvasc. Res. *21:* 267–298 (1981).
23 Weibel, E. R.: Morphometric estimation of pulmonary diffusion capacity. I. Model and method. Resp. Physiol. *11:* 54–75 (1970/1971).
24 Weibel, E. R.; Paumgartner, D.: Integrated stereological and biochemical studies on hepatocytic membranes. II. Correction of section thickness effect on volume and surface density estimates. J. Cell Biol. *77:* 584–597 (1978).
25 Weibel, E. R.: Practical methods for biological morphometry; in Weibel (ed.), Stereological methods, vol. 1 (Academic Press, New York 1979).

D. O. DeFouw, PhD, Department of Anatomy, UMDNJ-New Jersey Medical School, 100 Bergen Street, Newark, NJ 07103 (USA)

Prog. appl. Microcirc., vol. 9, pp. 80–87 (Karger, Basel 1985)

Discussion of the Presentations: *Clough, Schneeberger, DeFouw*

BERNAUDIN: I would like to discuss the role of junctions and vesicles in the microcirculation of the lung (showed 8 slides). We have used anti-HRP antibodies as a tracer, which is quite physiological, because it is an immunoglobulin. When detecting autologous antibodies in the rat lung, we found some of these throughout some interendothelial junctions. They were also seen in structures looking like channels, but these were quite rare in the lung. Most of the junctions, however, were not filled with the reaction product. After intravenous injection of heterologous or isologous IgG, they were detected in vesicles opening onto or close to the luminal surface. From 90 min to 16 h positive vesicles close to the basement membrane or close to the albuminal front were very rare, and the basement membrane was stained only after 24 h. When we used fragments such as FAB'2 or FAB (mol. weight 100,000 daltons) these tracers were observed on the abluminal side as early as 30 min for FAB'2 and 10 min for FAB. Several interendothelial junctions were filled continuously with the tracers, but only very few positive vesicles were observed in the cytoplasm of the endothelial cells. In addition, we also used this method to study the blood-brain barrier in the rat. We found an early detection of autologous antibodies in the brain capillaries but no IgG on the tissue front or on the basement membrane. Vescicles were for the most part rare and only close to the luminal side and junctions remained unstained. By contrast, in the choroid plexus the autologous IgG was detected in the epithelial basement membrane, in the tissue, and also in the intercellular clefts up to their tight junctions. In the mesothelium from rat parietal pleural we found autologous IgG, mainly in the intercellular junctions. Very few if any positive vesicles were detected and the positive vesicles were always close to the luminal or abluminal side or to the intercellular spaces. With this method we obtained no data which permits us to say that there is a transport by vesicles. Even for immunoglobulins, i.e., proteins, the junctions and not the vesicles appear to be an important route.

WILLIAMS: We are using an isolated capillary system to study endocytosis, i.e., the original part of vesicular transport, the endocytic sequestration of molecules. I look at endocytosis from the standpoint of two types of possible kinetics, either fluid phase kinetics or adsorptive phase kinetics. In fluid phase kinetics the relationship between the rate of endocytosis is strictly dependent upon the concentration of molecules outside. Since there is no interaction of the solute with the membrane, there is a direct linear relationship between the concentration of material and the rate of endocytosis. We would have expected in the past that most molecules in the plasma would follow these kinetics. There is another possibility and that is adsorptive phase endocytosis, which is a receptor-mediated endocytosis, but cationized ferritin can also follow adsorptive phase endocytosis. As there is an interaction of molecules with the membrane, we have a more complex kinetic analysis of this type of endocytosis. It is non-linear; it is dependent on the external concentration, but it is also dependent upon a number of other variables. This is demonstrated by two molecules that we have looked at and I will show you what sort of kinetics they follow. The first molecule is sucrose. If one looks at the relationship between external sucrose concentration and its ability to be sequestered by endothelial cells, one finds a strict linear relationship between one and a thousand micromolar external concentration. That makes a very good marker of fluid phase endocytosis with no interaction with the endothelial cell membrane. On the other hand, if we look at ferritin, a molecule that many of us have used for years as a marker of fluid phase endocytosis, we see that it obeys kinetics of adsorptive phase endocytosis, because ferritin is concentrated in the vesicles and it obeys a non-linear relationship. Native anionic ferritin (pH range 4.6 to 5) is sequestered within the vesicles. Albumin is essentially ecxluded from vesicular transport in a purified isolated capillary system. However, when we mix ferritin and albumin together in much the same way that Drs. BALDWIN, CLOUGH and SCHNEEBERGER have done in their glutaraldehyde fixed specimens, we find that albumin interferes with the sequestration of ferritin into vesicles. As we raise the albumin concentration in the external media, we find reduced binding and labelling of ferritin to the membrane. Regarding specificity, we find that in a purified system, purified albumin is excluded from vesicular transport. Therefore it is a rather poor molecule to study vesicular transport in endothelial cells. However, if we take albumin and glucosylate it, the relative extent of glucosylation is two molecules of glucose per molecule of albumin, we find a reversal of this exclusion. Glucosylated albumin is now vesicularly transported. Endothelial cells have receptors for certain molecules and this glucosylation has another dramatic effect: LDLs bind to the endothelial cell at 4 °C and they are endocytically sequestered with a difference between 37 °C and 4 °C. Following glucosylation of the LDL, glucose attacks the lysines on LDL, and there is a reduction in both the binding and a lack of endocytosis of the LDL molecule. Endocytosis of the LDL by the endothelial cell requires a very specifically placed lysine. If you block that lysine there is no endocytosis of LDL. This has been seen not only by us in capillary endothelial cells but by a number of other investigators in a number of other cellular systems. Morphological evidence for glucosylated protein and a glucosylated anionic protein can be shown with cultured endothelial cells. When the protein is non-glucosylated there is very little interaction with the endothelial cells. When it is glucosylated there is a rather dramatic change in this interaction.

MICHEL: I would like to comment on Dr. WILLIAMS' remarks. First of all, I am very concerned if he is actually looking at uptake into the same population of vesicles which dominate electron micrographs. The first reason for asking this question is that the time-course of uptake is very different from the time-course which Dr. CLOUGH showed, and which our group previously showed, for the approach to a steady state of labelling during ferritin perfusion in frog endothelium. The second reason is the preferential uptake of ferritin. When one examines electron micrographs of ferritin molecules inside vesicles, ferritin appears to be excluded, far away beyond the steric exclusion you would expect between spherical ferritin molecules and the bare walls of the vesicular cavities, to an extent that half or even more of the vesicular volume must be occupied by something else because less than half of it is actually available to the ferritin molecules. So the morphological evidence is that the ferritin is excluded. The third point is related to the fact that the distribution of ferritin molecules within vesicles followed a *Poisson* distribution, indicating that the native ferritin molecules were distributed as by chance. There appeared to be no particular mechanism other than random movements of the ferritin into the luminal vesicular cavities.

WILLIAMS: The time-course concerns that you have, I and others are well aware that using the isolated system our time-course is much longer. But I'd like to suggest that time-course is relative to the isolated system and there are a couple of other differences. First of all, our endothelial cells have a slightly increased number of vesicles and their luminal and abluminal distances are slightly larger. That would increase the time necessary for the vesicles to move inside the cell. The other point is that the time to achieve biochemical equilibration differs between molecules, but for the most part it takes up to 30–40 min to reach 100% equilibration. Morphologically, one is never completely sure when equilibration is reached, because the difference between 95% vesicular filling and 100% vesicular filling is not as clear morphologically. Regarding our time-course for a number of molecules, we see 60–70% filling of the vesicles within 4–5 min after the molecules start associating with these endothelial cells. So there is an initial rapid phase of filling. The problem is that it is much like a bus system. You can pick up the first few passengers very quickly, but to get them all crowded on takes a little bit of rearrangement.

MICHEL: That's still an order of magnitude lower that what we found. We're seeing equilibration or near steady state in 45 s.

WILLIAMS: When you say equilibrium are you talking about 100% filling?

MICHEL: No, steady state.

WAGNER: I'd like to make a comment about orders of magnitude here in your so-called kinctic studies. We're looking at an average of about 140,000 endothelial cells for each one of those points on there. The kinetic studies that are done here compared to electron micrographs, I would think would be performed on an infinitesimally smaller sample size than the information that is presented on those graphs.

WILLIAMS: I'd like to address the two other points that Dr. MICHEL raised. The difficulty in working with ferritin is the type of molecule we are dealing with. Ferritin ranges as far as the extent of glucosylation is concerned anywhere from 40–50% down to 0%. So your results depend on the type of ferritin you're using. If you're recrystallizing ferritin a number of times, you find that it is non-glucosylated and in our hands ferritin with no glucosylation is excluded from vesicles. That problem must be cleared up methodologically. Regarding the distributions, we are talking unfortunately about the difference between biochemical and morphological analyses and that is going to take a little bit of time to work out.

WILLIAMSON: There are two comments I'd like to make. One relates to the point Dr. CLOUGH made on the fixative effects on the thickness of endothelium in the mesenteric capillaries. I believe it was about half as thick with glutaraldehyde as it was with the osmium fixation and she suggested that perhaps glutaraldehyde induces shrinking of the endothelium. The point I would like to make is whether osmium induces swelling or glutaraldehyde shrinking? I think osmolarity of the fixative is probably far more important than the fixative agent itself. I was struck also by the fact that there appeared to be a little difference in endothelial thickness in the electron micrographs that Dr. CASLEY-SMITH and Dr. FRØKJÆR-JENSEN have shown to us. But I think that swelling of endothelium could indeed cause marked artifacts in the apparent distribution of vesicles and that may really be the crux of the problem with fixation. The other comment is to Dr. SCHNEEBERGER's presentation. I was very much struck with her results found in fetal lamb vs. mature lamb: Very few vesicles in the fetal animal and very striking numbers of them in the mature lamb. This brings to mind a study that we did years ago on a cell which contains perhaps the most microvesicles of any cell in the body, perhaps most analogous to the endothelium and has not yet been mentioned this morning, and that is the lipid-depleted fat cell. If you look at a normal fat cell which is full of lipid, you see just occasional vesicles, just as Dr. SCHNEEBERGER showed us in the fetal capillary of the lung. But if you starve the rat for various periods of time, but up to the point that it loses 30–40% of its body weight, the cytoplasm of the fat cell becomes absolutely filled with microvesicles and invaginations of the plasma membrane that are indistinguishable from those of the endothelium. The point I would emphasize here is that there is no reason to think that those microvesicles are at all concerned with the transport of macromolecules.

CRONE: I have a question to Dr. SCHNEEBERGER's very interesting presentation. Are we learning now that albumin is not transported by vesicular transport? If we are learning that, then to me the world is really upside down, because the vesicular system according to *Palade* and almost all of us is designed to transport plasma proteins, more than half of which is albumin. Are we now learning that it is there to transport ferritin?

SCHNEEBERGER: I hope I didn't give you that impression. I wanted to see what effect circulating proteins have on the marker molecule, another macromolecule. As I showed yesterday, as opposed to some of my colleagues here, I find very nice immunocytochemical evidence of albumin in vesicles. I just wanted to point out that the world is right side up. But I want also to emphasize that the system I use is a rather tricky one, because

I'm using lyophilized rat serum protein and, as you know, albumin is one of the few serum proteins which is predominantly non-glucosylated. Immunoglobulins and all the rest are glucosylated and there is the phenomenon of piggy-back, where glucosylated molecules actually complex with non-glucosylated ones. So I don't know how the albumin got into the vesicles. I think Dr. WILLIAMS works with an absolutely pure system. I'm using lyophilized rat serum protein with a whole spectrum of proteins, but I'm actually localizing individual proteins by immunocytochemical means, by antibodies to albumin or immunoglobulin G. It may well be that other molecules may actually be carrying the albumin for all I know.

RIPPE: If we accept that the vesicular system can not only transport ferritin, but may take up albumin after all, studies we made in the middle of the 70's where we cooled down endothelium indicated that the transport processes for albumin were totally passive. Another aspect of that work is that we found a correlation between the colloid oncotic pressure gradient over the capillary membrane and the transport of albumin during isogravimetry. The only theory which can account for such a transport is transport through small and large pores, where the bulk of the albumin is going through a large pore system. This could be either chains of fused vesicles, but these studies indicated that dissipative mechanisms could be responsible for only a very, very small fraction of the transport through the endothelium.

WILLIAMS: Let me make a comment as far as the albumin is concerned. We are dealing with, as Dr. SCHNEEBERGER said, a highly purified system of capillaries and a highly purified system of albumin, where we take 100% non-glucosylated albumin and put it in with purified cells and it is excluded. In the body albumin exists as approximately 10% glucosylated and 90% non-glucosylated. I would certainly expect with our biochemical data that we find both of these forms of albumin glucosylated and non-glucosylated in vesicles. Dr. SCHNEEBERGER also finds albumin within the vesicles, immunocytochemically, and I would suggest that a large proportion of that albumin is in the glucosylated form and indeed when we test lymph we find in it a preferential existence of glucosylated albumin as well as in the urine of even normal animals. There is a preference for the glucosylated form of albumin, but that does not mean that non-glucosylated albumin is excluded in the normal functioning individual. It is carried with the glucosylated albumin and quite possibly by other serum proteins.

J. RYAN: How strong is this preference? It is 10% in the plasma: what is it in the lymph?

WILLIAMS: If you look in the plasma of a normal individual it is about 10%. If you look in kidney lymph it is about 40-45%.

U. RYAN: I'd like to follow up on the point Dr. WILLIAMSON made in interpreting Dr. SCHNEEBERGER's sequence in the fetal lamb. There is a completely different explanation one could arrive at and that is, that in the fetal lamb there is very little processing of circulating vasoactive substances, whereas in the adult lamb there is an activity I certainly don't question. One could look at the vesicles in those terms, without ever worrying about these other issues.

SCHNEEBERGER: Just to follow up on that. When I wrote the paper I actually referred very much to *Alex Stallcup*'s work, where he showed very nicely that these surface enzymes on endothelium increase with gestational time. I think that explanation is also perfectly valid. It could also explain the dearth of vesicles early in gestation.

WAYLAND: I think we are getting a little confused here between endocytosis and transcytosis. In the first place the best evidence that I know is that molecules as big as serum albumin are not transported across capillary walls. Most of the serum albumin gets across on the venular side and we have different structures, which we really haven't explored in this meaning. Actually the evidence of transport is relatively small compared to the evidence of being picked up by the vesicles. I think we have to recognize that there is a real difference between these. Also in connection with the LDL we found in vivo that at least tagged LDL was indeed sequestered by endothelial cells in the rat mesentery. We also found that VLDL was sequestered. HDL was not, and it does not carry any glycoproteins nor is it acted on by the normal receptors for the LDL. Also the gamma globulin was sequestered. In every case where there was glycoprotein present, we found sequestration. However, we found no sequestration, in the case of serum albumin, and in the case of HDL. Here we're talking about endocytosis, not transcytosis.

HAMMERSEN: Are you referring to the so-called gradient of vascular permeability?

WAYLAND: I'm talking about the very specific evidence that most of the transport of the large molecules takes place on the venular side and not at the capillary. It isn't a simple gradient.

HAMMERSEN: Everybody agrees with you, but the endothelium of this side is almost identically organized. There might be some fenestrations, but I don't think from a structural point of view that there is such a tremendous difference between an endothelium of a venule or a true capillary, whatever true capillary means.

WAYLAND: But how about the junction?

HAMMERSEN: There might be a difference in the junctions, but as far as I know there is not much evidence that albumin is passing through junctions.

MICHEL: I don't know if Dr. RENKIN is here, because he is the person to make the point.

RENKIN: I didn't want to address that. I had my hand up for another reason. I wanted to challenge Dr. WAYLAND's statement that all physiologists believe that large molecules are exchanged preferentially in the venules. I don't believe it. As time has gone on the number of visible dye leaks that people have recorded from the venules in microvascular preparations has got smaller and smaller. Now one finds in the literature one to three leaks in a good resting preparation per square millimeter. In a square millimeter there are something of the order of a hundred capillaries and if you calculate the hypothetical large pore system, there are couple of hundred large pores in that system. So they are not identical with the leaks. The leaks in the resting state represent one or two percent of the large pore system and therefore have to be considered as a supplementary still larger pore system that is present in a very low level, but is not sufficient to account for the movement of say albumin or other proteins in the resting state. As far as the albumin goes there are some problems with evaluating the magnitude of the large pore system. It is possible that all of the albumin could be accounted for by going through large pores. It is also possible that the large pores are not sufficient to account for the albumin so that a part of it goes through some other system, which may be vesicular. But the real problem is evaluating how much of the fluid movement goes through the large pore system and how much albumin it would carry. I think this question is still open.

END OF DISCUSSION

Prog. appl. Microcirc., vol. 9, pp. 88–99 (Karger, Basel 1985)

The Study of Endothelial Vesicles in the Isolated Perfused Lymphatic Vessel

C. C. C. O'Morchoe[a], *H. M. Jarosz*[b], *W. R. Jones*[b], *P. J. O'Morchoe*[a]

[a] Departments of Anatomy and Pathology, University of Illinois, College of Medicine at Urbana-Champaign, Urbana, Ill., USA

[b] Departments of Anatomy and Pathology, Loyola University of Chicago, Stritch School of Medicine, Maywood, Ill., USA

Introduction

An endocytotic vesicular system is a characteristic component of endothelial cells whether they be lymphatic or blood vascular in nature. Despite this ubiquity, there is much that is as yet unknown about the structure of the system and about its role in molecular transport to or from the lumen of the vessel. Experimental evidence exists to indicate that, in the case of blood capillary endothelium, vesicles are of prime importance in the exodus of plasma proteins from vessel lumen to interstitium [2, 6]. According to this view, the vesicular system is largely composed of discrete vesicles, derived from caveolae which form upon the luminal face and shuttle to the interstitial surface of the cell, there to release their contents. Disagreement with this viewpoint is based on several factors, one of which is that vesicles may not exist as discrete cytoplasmic entities, but form instead, a system of interconnecting spheres and channels. Ultrastructural observations consistent with this latter viewpoint have been reported [3].

Comparable considerations pertain to the vesicular system of lymphatic endothelium, although here it may be expected that, if a transport role exists, it will function in the opposite direction – that is, from interstitium to lumen. Analysis of transport across lymphatic endothelium in vivo is technically difficult and has, therefore, been confined to such sites as the diaphragm [7], where lymphatics drain the peritoneal cavity. The lymphatic vessels at that site are relatively accessible for structural studies using visible tracers, when compared to deeper sites within the organs and other tissues of the body. However, because of the effect of respiratory movements, the mechanism of transport into lymph across lymphatic endothelium in specialized areas, such as the diaphragm, is almost certainly quite different from that in other regions of the body.

The inaccessibility of most lymphatic vessels to transport studies, has led us to develop a technique applicable to isolated perfused lymphatic vessels. Such a preparation permits measurement of the rate at which substances cross the lymphatic wall from bathing fluid to vessel lumen as well as in the opposite direction. In addition, it enables the isolated vessel wall to be fixed rapidly at the end of the experiment. This rapidity with which fixation is achieved also makes the technique suitable for ultrastructural tracer studies to illustrate the transport pathways. This report describes the procedures that we use, presents results obtained from studies using horseradish peroxidase as a tracer, and discusses some of the advantages and problems inherent in the methodology.

Material and Methods

Segments of renal hilar lymphatics were isolated from dogs and transferred to a chamber containing Delbecco's Modified Eagles Medium (DMEM). There they were perfused with DMEM before horseradish peroxidase (HRP) was added to either the bathing or perfusion fluid. Karnovsky's fixative was then substituted for the bathing fluid and the lymphatics processed for electron microscopy.

Isolation and Perfusion of Lymphatic Segments

Mongrel dogs of either sex were anesthetized with intravenous sodium pentobarbital and then subjected to a left loin incision for exposure of the renal pedicle. The tissues covering and adjoining the posterior aspect of the pedicle were examined through a Zeiss binocular microscope for lymphatic vessels belonging to the renal hilar system. Typically, a lymph node lies towards the medial end of the pedicle on its caudal aspect, and into this node drain two or three small vessels from the renal hilus. These vessels were sought first, and, when present, were isolated in turn and used experimentally. The next lymphatics to be prepared were those that lay in close association with the renal artery, and finally, lymphatics lying parallel and rostral to the renal artery and vein were used.

After the lymphatics on the left side had been prepared and studied, the animal was turned over and the right renal pedicle exposed for similar lymphatic isolation. On both sides, only one lymphatic was isolated and cannulated at a time, the remainder being left as undisturbed as possible until they in turn were isolated. Typically two to six lymphatic segments on either side of each animal were successfully isolated, cannulated and perfused.

Each segment consisted of a variable length of the lymphatic that was free of branches or tributaries. It was dissected cleanly, cannulated with polyethylene tubing (PELO) at each end (fig. 1), and separated from the rest of the lymphatic. The segment with the two cannulae in place was then supported, to prevent its kinking while in transit, and transferred to a perfusion chamber containing DMEM. The inflow cannula was connected to the outflow from a Sage syringe-type pump, which was set to deliver DMEM at about 2 μl/min through the lymphatic segment. The outflow cannula was drained by touching it to a 10 μl glass pipette. The perfusion chamber contained a built-in heating element, which was regulated with the aid of a thermocouple, to keep the bathing fluid at a constant temperature (37 °C). The fluid was also controlled for pH and was stirred and oxygenated with a bubbling system. Each lymphatic segment was perfused with DMEM (2 μl/min) for 5 min to remove retained lymph protein from its lumen before the addition of tracer.

Four main groups of lymphatic segments were studied. In one group of five segments HRP, in a concentration of 0.03 g%, was maintained in the bathing fluid for 1 min prior to fixation. In a second group of six segments, HRP in the same concentration was added to the perfusion fluid for a 1-min-period before fixation. The third group of four lymphatics served as a control for the first two, being treated and processed in the same manner but without the addition of HRP to either bathing or perfusion fluid. In the fourth group of 17 lymphatic

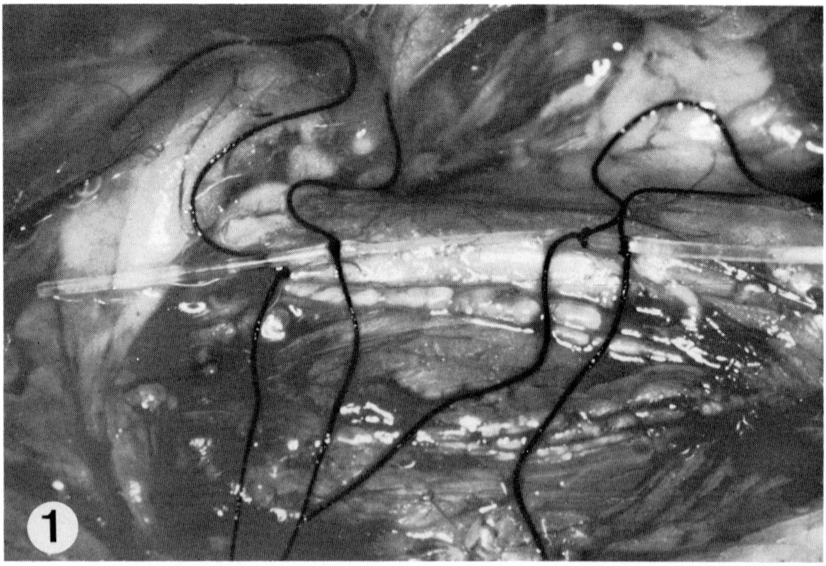

Fig. 1. Photograph of a typical renal hilar lymphatic segment, as used in the present study, before removal from the animal. An inflow and an outflow cannula are tied in place. The transparency of the lymphatic walls is evident because vasa vasorum of the renal artery can be seen through them.

segments, HRP was added to the bathing fluid in a concentration of 3.0 g% for intervals of 5, 15, and 30 s and 1, 5 and 10 min prior to fixation.

Tissue Preparation and Examination

Immediately upon completion of the exposure to HRP, the bathing fluid was changed to Karnovsky's fixative (4 °C) and the lymphatic disconnected and maintained in additional cold Karnovsky's fixative overnight. It was then rinsed in cacodylate buffer before the HRP reaction was induced with diaminobenzidine (DAB). Thereafter, the tissue was rinsed, osmicated for 30 min and dehydrated in acetone, before being embedded in Epon and sectioned (fig. 2). Thin sections for electron microscopy were stained lightly with bismuth.

Electron micrographs were examined for the integrity of the endothelial wall, the quality of the fixation and the presence of HRP reaction product in the endothelial cells. Preparations, which revealed reaction product apparently free within the cytoplasm, were discarded, although this finding was rare. Only lymphatics, which showed the reaction product confined to the vesicular system or the intercellular pathways, were retained for data collection. In such vessels, the percentage of vesicles containing HRP reaction product (i. e., labeled) was determined not only for the endothelium as a whole but also according to the position of the vesicles in the cytoplasm. Thus, four vesicular groups were recognized

(1) showing attachment to the luminal membrane (L),
(2) showing attachment to the abluminal membrane (A),
(3) apparently lying free within the luminal half of the cytoplasm (CL), and
(4) apparently lying free within the abluminal half of the cytoplasm (AL).

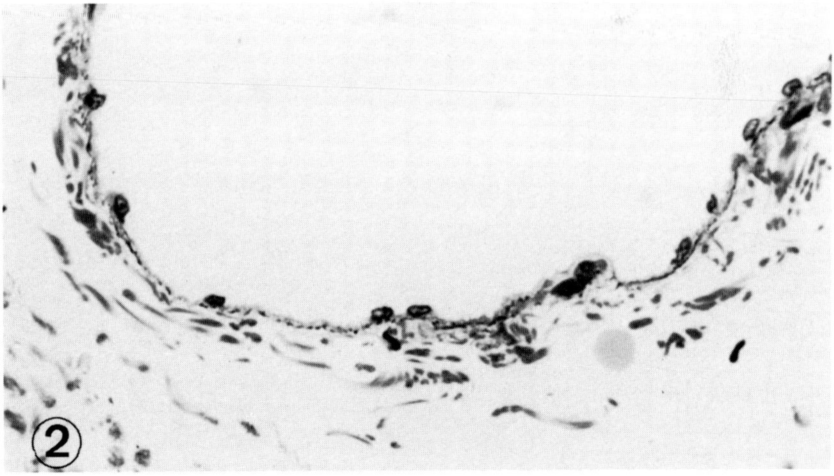

Fig. 2. Light micrograph of a renal lymphatic segment cut transversely. The vessel wall consists of a continuous thin endothelial lining and some loose connective tissue containing only occasional fibroblasts and smooth muscle cells.

Results

The lymphatic segments used in this study showed excellent preservation as judged by their general ultrastructural appearance and by the distribution of HRP within the cells. Only rarely was the HRP reaction product seen to lie free within the cytoplasm, and, since this was taken as evidence of cell damage, those specimens were discarded. In the overwhelming majority of lymphatic segments, the HRP reaction product was confined to the vesicular system and to the regions between cells.

Figure 3 is an example of a control lymphatic segment; that is, one untreated with HRP yet processed in the routine manner for the peroxidase reaction. It can be seen that the vesicular system contains little or no electron dense material. In contrast, figure 4 reveals the intense reaction product that pervades the endocytotic vesicular system when HRP has been added to the bathing fluid before fixation. A consistent finding, also portrayed in figure 4 was that the luminal vesicles and luminal membrane showed a more intense concentration of reaction product than did the

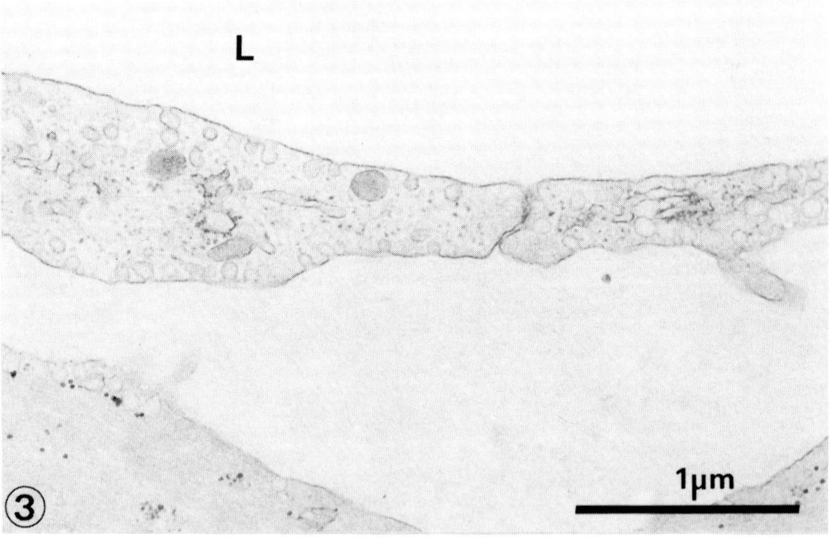

Fig. 3. Electron micrograph of a control lymphatic segment processed in the routine manner, but without the addition of HRP at any time. This and other sections were stained with bismuth only. The endocytotic vesicular system contains little or no electron dense material. *L* = Lumen; magnification × 31,000.

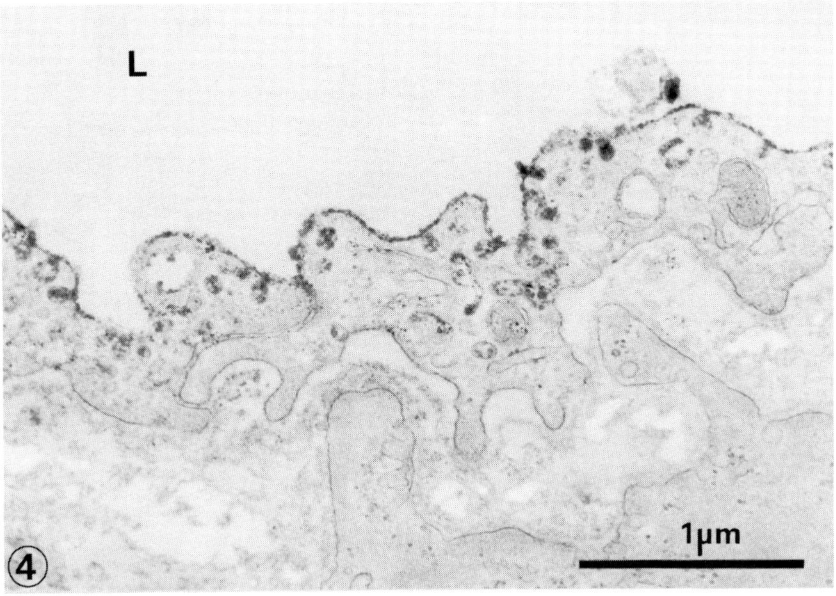

Fig. 4. Electron micrograph of a lymphatic segment after HRP had been added to the bathing fluid (thus applied abluminally) for 10 min at a concentration of 3.0 g%. The HRP reaction product can be seen through the endocytotic vesicular system. The intensity of the reaction product is much greater on the luminal membrane and in the luminal vesicles than on the abluminal membrane, abluminal vesicles or even the interstitium, thus suggesting a binding or concentration phenomenon. *L* = Lumen; magnification × 31,000.

abluminal region, even when the HRP was given abluminally. Thus, it was evident from these specimens that HRP rapidly traversed the thickness of the endothelium, from abluminal to luminal surface, through the vesicular system. In contrast, when HRP was added to the perfusion fluid, and thus was presented only to the luminal membrane, it remained confined to those vesicles in direct contact with the luminal surface, or those so closely related to it that they may have opened to the surface out of the plane of section. In no instance was HRP seen to travel through the vesicular system from lumen to abluminal surface.

The quantitative data on the distribution of HRP labeled vesicles are shown in figures 5 (abluminal application) and 6 (luminal application). They corroborate the qualitative observations described above. Additional data pertaining to the speed with which HRP traversed the vesicular system is shown in figure 7. It can be seen that 90% of vesicles attached to

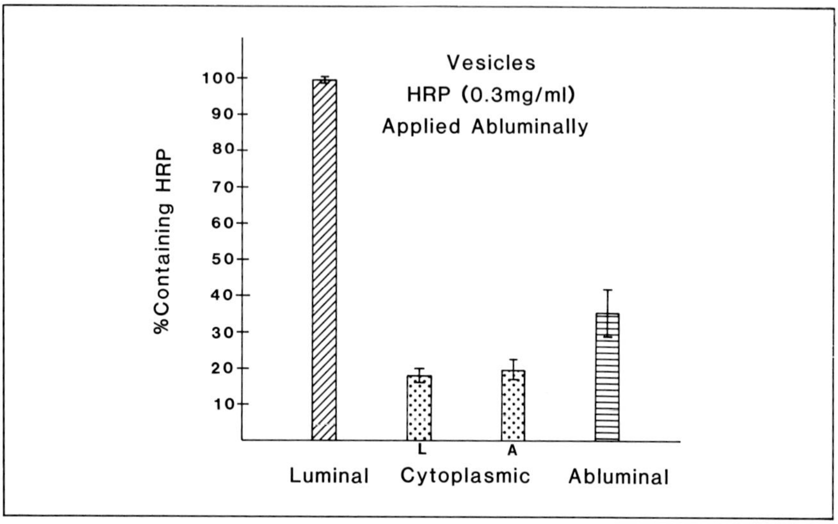

Fig. 5. Histogram showing the percentage of vesicles labeled after the abluminal application (in the bathing fluid) of HRP, according to their position in the endothelial cells (*L* = luminal half of cytoplasm; *A* = abluminal half of cytoplasm).

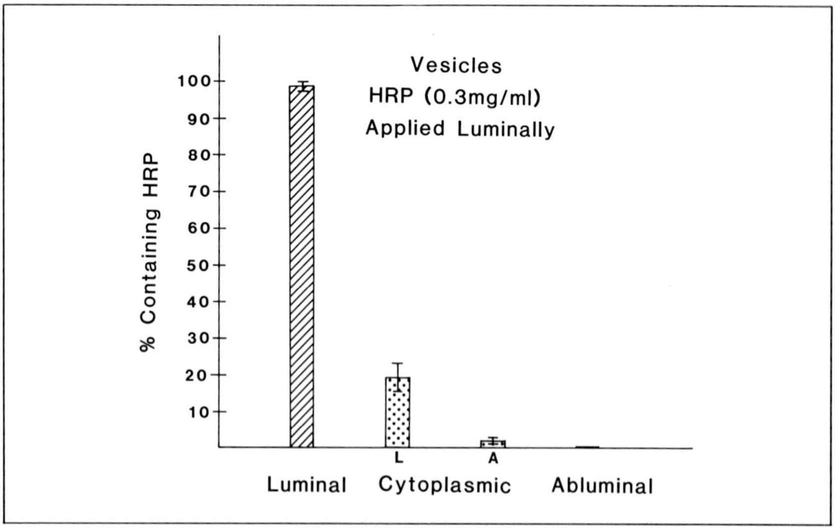

Fig. 6. Histogram showing the percentage of vesicles labeled after the luminal application (in the perfusion fluid) of HRP, according to their position in the endothelial cells (*L* = luminal half of cytoplasm; *A* = abluminal half of cytoplasm).

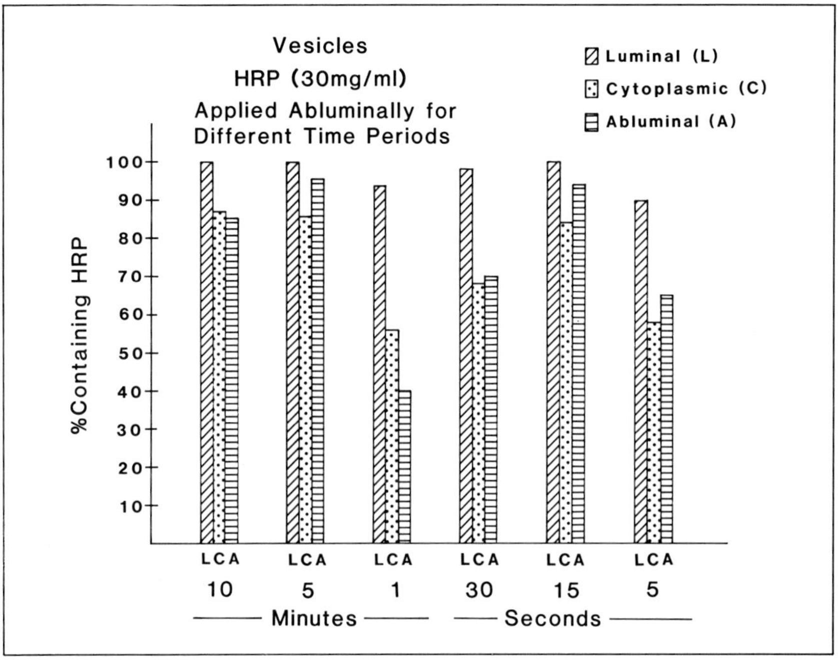

Fig. 7. Histogram showing the percentage of labeled vesicles after the abluminal application (in the bathing fluid) of HRP, according to their position in the endothelial cells. The times indicated on the abscissa denote the length of exposure of the lymphatic segment to HRP.

the luminal membrane were labeled even when fixation was started within 5 s of the application of HRP to the abluminal lymphatic wall. After 15 s approximately 100% of luminal vesicles were labeled. One somewhat surprising finding, seen in figures 5 and 7, was that a higher percentage of luminal than abluminal vesicles was labeled, even when the HRP was applied to the abluminal endothelial face. We believe that this is related to the unexplained greater concentration of reaction product at the luminal face, which made the presence of label in luminal vesicles more obvious.

Discussion

We consider that the technique utilized in this study, whereby lymphatic vessels are isolated and studied in vitro, can provide valuable information on transendothelial transport. It provides the only known model in which the rate of movement of substances across the lymphatic endothelial wall can be examined free from the influence of the blood capillary wall. It also lends itself to ultrastructural tracer studies of transport pathways because of the rapidity with which tissue fixation can be achieved. However, considerations of the validity of data generated by the technique raise questions that need to be addressed here.

One such question is, whether the lymphatic segments retain their integrity or viability during the course of the experiments. The present observations, as well as those from a previous study in our laboratory [5], clearly indicate that they do. Three lines of evidence may be cited. One is that the ultrastructure of the endothelium, after as long as 90 min perfusion in vitro, is qualitatively and quantitatively indistinguishable from control lymphatic endothelium fixed in vivo [5]. Second, the rate of protein movement across the endothelium in vitro, under static conditions, is relatively consistent among different lymphatic segments and is quite constant for any one lymphatic during a 90 min experiment [5]. The third is that HRP, when administered in the bathing or perfusion fluid, is confined in almost all specimens to the endocytotic vesicular system and to the regions between the cells (fig. 4). Damaged cells, on the other hand, show HRP diffusely spread throughout the cytoplasm.

A second question concerns the type of lymphatic vessels used in the present study. These, by definition, must be regarded as collecting vessels and thus may differ from initial vessels both in their function and in the thickness of their wall. Ultrastructurally, however, the endothelium of canine renal hilar vessels is comparable to that of intrarenal lymphatics that are associated with the lobules of the cortex [1]. These latter are the initial lymph-forming vessels of the kidney, which have also been shown to have HRP in their vesicular system after the tracer has been added to the general circulation in living animals.

A second point of major relevance to this question is that dogs have unusually thin-walled collecting lymphatic vessels. Figure 2 illustrates this point: The wall of a typical hilar vessel is shown. It comprises only an endothelial lining and some loose connective tissue, which contains occasional scattered fibroblasts and smooth muscle cells. Indeed, the thickness of this wall is little different from that of the interlobular lymphatics in the kidney, where the majority of renal lymph is considered to be formed. Interestingly, comparable hilar lymphatic vessels in the rat, for instance, have thicker walls containing two or three continuous layers of muscle cells, and thus are more consistent with the usual description of collecting vessels. The reason for this species difference is not known. The speed – a matter of seconds – with which HRP crossed from the bathing fluid to the luminal membrane of the endothelium in the present study, confirms that the extra-endothelial elements of the canine renal hilar lymphatic do not constitute a barrier to the movement of this tracer.

A third major question is, whether lymphatic endothelium, under the conditions of our experiment, behaves like endothelium in the living animal – at least as far as transport is concerned. The answer is clearly no, because the experiments performed so far have been deliberately carried out under static conditions in order that the behavior of the endothelium could be examined free of other influences such as hydrostatic and osmotic pressure, which are known to play a major role in lymph formation in vivo. However, in future studies our technique can be modified, with the aid of a suitable chamber, to simulate the effects of hydrostatic and osmotic influences on endothelial transport. We believe that the results of the present study reveal transendothelial movement of macromolecules even in the absence of external mechanical forces.

A final question is especially relevant to this study. It is, whether the endocytotic vesicular system of lymphatic endothelium comprises a more or less continuous interconnecting system that spans in toto or in part the endothelial cells, or whether it is a system of relatively discrete vesicles that move across the endothelium. This question applies to blood as well as to lymphatic endothelium and has not yet been satisfactorily resolved. The evidence suggests [4] that in lymphatic endothelium at least, the majority of vesicles (80–90%) are open to one or other surface, but not both, at any given time. The importance of this issue to the present study pertains to the manner in which the HRP can cross the cells. If the vesicular system is a continuous system, then HRP could cross from one surface to the other by simple diffusion. Alternatively, if continuous channels do not connect opposing surfaces, then some form of cytoplasmic process involved in membrane separation and fusion must occur for HRP to reach the lumen from the bathing fluid. Evidence derived from measurements of protein transport at different temperatures suggests that a cytoplasmic process is involved [5].

The role of intercellular channels in macromolecular transport is more difficult to assess in the present study. Reaction product was commonly seen between adjacent endothelial cells but often this appeared to be restricted by junctional complexes. Thus, although the evidence was not definitive, it did suggest that HRP could gain entrance to the lumen through the intercellular pathways. Movement in the opposite direction, from lumen to interstitium, was clearly impeded, if not prevented altogether. Therefore, it was concluded that the transport of HRP across the endothelium was governed by unidirectional forces. The nature of these forces is not clear, but is suggestive of a charge or binding phenomenon since HRP decorated the luminal membrane and vesicles much more intensely than their abluminal counterparts. This interpretation is consistent with other recent evidence from our laboratory (unpublished), using charged dyes and tracers, which indicates that there is a charge assymmetry between the two lymphatic endothelial surfaces.

Consideration of these various questions leads us to the conclusion that transport of HRP in vitro, as depicted in this study, reflects to some extent its transport in the living animal. If this assessment is correct, the present data are indicative of three conclusions:

(1) that HRP traverses the lymphatic wall through the vesicular system in an adluminal direction,

(2) that it does so very rapidly – within a matter of seconds, and

(3) that HRP does not cross the endothelium in the reverse direction, from lumen to interstitium.

Summary

The endocytotic vesicular system in lymphatic endothelium was examined for a macromolecular transport role using horseradish peroxidase (HRP) as a tracer. Canine renal hilar lymphatic vessels were isolated and cannulated in situ and then transferred to a perfusion chamber which was maintained under constant conditions. The inflow cannula was connected to a perfusion pump and the outflow cannula to a glass pipette so that the perfusion fluid and bathing fluid were separated from each other by the lymphatic wall. HRP, at a concentration of 0.03 g%, was added to either the bathing fluid or the perfusion fluid for 10 min prior to rapid fixation and removal of the tissue. In another group of lymphatic segments, HRP was added to the bathing fluid at a concentration of 3.0 g%, for intervals of 5, 15 and 30 s and 1, 5, and 10 min prior to fixation. The percentage of vesicles containing HRP, classified according to their position in the cell, was then counted in electron micrographs. The data indicate that

(1) HRP traverses the lymphatic wall through the vesicular system in an adluminal direction,

(2) it does so very rapidly – within a matter of seconds, and

(3) HRP does not cross the endothelium in the reverse direction, from lumen to interstitium.

References

1 Albertine, K. H.; O'Morchoe, C. C. C.: Renal lymphatic ultrastructure and translymphatic transport. Microvasc. Res. *19:* 338–351 (1980).
2 Bruns, R. R.; Palade, G. E.: Studies on blood capillaries. I. General organization of blood capillaries in muscle. J. Cell Biol. *37:* 244–276 (1968).
3 Bundgaard, M.; Hagman, P.; Crone, C.: The three-dimensional organization of plasmalemmal vesicular profiles in the endothelium of rat heart capillaries. Microvasc. Res. *25:* 358–368 (1983).
4 Jones, W. R.; O'Morchoe, P. J.; O'Morchoe, C. C. C.: The organization of endocytotic vesicles in lymphatic endothelium. Microvasc. Res. *25:* 286–299 (1983).
5 O'Morchoe, C. C. C.; Jones III, W. R.; Jarosz, H. M.; O'Morchoe, P. J.; Fox, L. M.: Temperature dependence of protein transport across lymphatic endothelium in vitro. J. Cell Biol. *98:* 629–640 (1984).
6 Palade, G. E.; Bruns, R. R.: Structural modulations of plasmalemmal vesicles. J. Cell Biol. *37:* 633–649 (1968).
7 Tsilibary, E. C.; Wissig, S. L.: Absorption from the peritoneal cavity: SEM study of the mesothelium, covering the peritoneal surface of the muscular portion of the diaphragm. Am. J. Anat. *149:* 127–133 (1977).

C. C. C. O'Morchoe, MD, PhD, DSc, Department of Anatomy, University of Illinois, College of Medicine at Urbana-Champaign, 190 Medical Sciences Building, 506 South Mathews, Urbana, IL 61801 (USA)

Prog. appl. Microcirc., vol. 9, pp. 100–115 (Karger, Basel 1985)

Use of Lymphatic Protein Fluxes to Assess Vascular Endothelial Selectivity to Macromolecules

A. E. Taylor, R. J. Korthuis[a], *M. I. Townsley*[a]

Department of Physiology, College of Medicine, University of South Alabama, Mobile, Ala., USA

[a] Parker B. Francis Fellows of the Puritan-Bennett Foundation

Introduction

For several years physiologists have attempted to understand how large molecules leave the circulation and gain access to the interstitium, to finally be removed by the lymphatic system [8]. The classical studies of *Grotte* [11] and *Mayerson* et al. [13] analyzed lymph concentrations of various sized dextrans in different organs and showed differences between transcapillary exchange rates and a definite size selectivity, indicating that molecules with radii greater than about 45 Å do not cross most microcirculatory endothelial barriers to any great degree. The concept of how macromolecules crossed the microcirculation lay rather dormant until the late 1970's when *Renkin*'s [19, 20] and other studies [4, 18, 23, 24] stimulated several groups to begin to reassess the usage of lymph protein fluxes to measure microvascular permeability to plasma proteins [1–3, 6, 10, 14, 22, 25–28]. The purpose of this presentation is to describe how lymph can be used to estimate the permeability characteristics of the microvascular walls to the passage of macromolecules across its boundaries, and how these macromolecule permeability estimates can be used to describe the endothelial barrier.

Mathematical Models

For many years it was thought that the flux of a protein (J_s) could be explained by the linear *Kedem and Katchalsky* [12] equation:

$$J_s = (1-\sigma)\,\overline{C}_s J_v + PS\Delta C_s \qquad (1)$$

where σ is the reflection coefficient of the macromolecule, $\overline{C}_s$ is its average concentration, J_v is the amount of capillary filtration occuring, PS is the permeability coefficient-surface area product and ΔC_s is the concentration gradient of the macromolecule existing between plasma (C_P) and the interstitium (C_T).

We used this equation to evaluate σ and PS for plasma proteins by collecting lymph from an organ at two different lymph flow rates and solving the two resulting equations when J_v, J_s (equals $J_v \cdot C_T$), $\overline{C}_s$ and ΔC_s are measured for each flow state [24]. To our surprise, σ and PS were functions of lymph flow (or capillary filtration rate) and were not constants for a given solute-solvent-system as required by equation 1. Although several physiological properties could cause this abberant phenomenological result, we noted that when capillary filtration was extremely high a solution was possible [3]. But, it remained for *Rutili* et al. [22] to point out that the problem in using equation 1 is that it does not describe the fluxes associated with filtration occuring across a membrane, unless PSΔC approaches zero at high volume fluxes.

The equation used by *Granger and Taylor* [10] which was adapted from the *Patlak* equation [17] describes how the filtrate relative to filtrand behaves as the amount of filtration increases. If we perceive the capillary ultrafiltrate as the lymph concentration of a macromolecule (C_L) and the filtrand as the plasma concentration (C_P), then:

$$C_L/C_P = \frac{1-\sigma}{1-\sigma e^{-x}} \qquad (2)$$

where $x = (1-\sigma)J_v/PS$. (3)

When the lymph flow is large, C_L/C_P approaches $1-\sigma$ and we have a unique means of assessing a selectivity factor of the macromolecule at the membrane interface – σ, the reflection coefficient.

Figure 1 shows how C_L/C_P behaves when lymph flow is increased by elevating capillary pressure. For curve 1, $\sigma = 0.9$, and for curve 2, $\sigma = 0.7$. Note that at high J_v, $C_L/C_P \rightarrow 1-\sigma$ for both cases, i.e., 0.1 and 0.3, respectively. Also shown is a case when $\sigma = 0.9$ but surface area is doubled (line 3). C_L/C_P still will approach $1-\sigma$ but it will require a very high lymph flow. The importance of figure 1 is that one cannot simply look

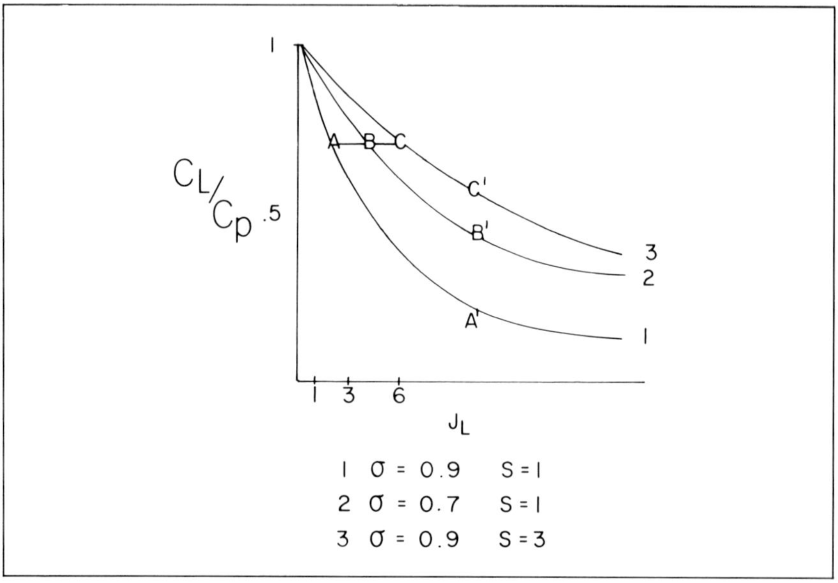

Fig. 1. Schematic plot of the protein concentration in lymph (C_L) relative to plasma (C_P) as lymph flow or capillary filtration is increased. Curves 1, 2, and 3 were constructed using the σs and surface areas shown on the legend. A^l, B^l, and C^l and A, B, and C are explained in the text (from [28], with permission).

at C_L/C_P for a given lymph flow (A^l, B^l, C^l) and use that information to evaluate the permeability properties of the endothelial barrier. Also, the same C_L/C_P can be obtained at very different lymph flows (A, B, C) either due to changes in vascular permeability or surface area [28]. Figure 1 shows that we can determine a unique σ but only if C_L/C_P is a constant; at other values, it is impossible to evaluate the permeability properties of the membrane.

Figure 2 shows how we can measure the selectivity of the microvascular wall to macromolecules [10, 22, 25–28]. First, C_L/C_P must become filtration independent before one can estimate σ. So, lymph flow must be elevated by increasing capillary pressure until a constant C_L/C_P is obtained. When that occurs, a unique σ is obtained for any given macromolecule which is contained in both lymph and plasma.

Figure 3 A, B, and C show lymph to plasma ratios of different sized macromolecules in lymph and plasma as a function of molecular radius for these different vascular beds. Note that a precipitous fall in C_L (or L)

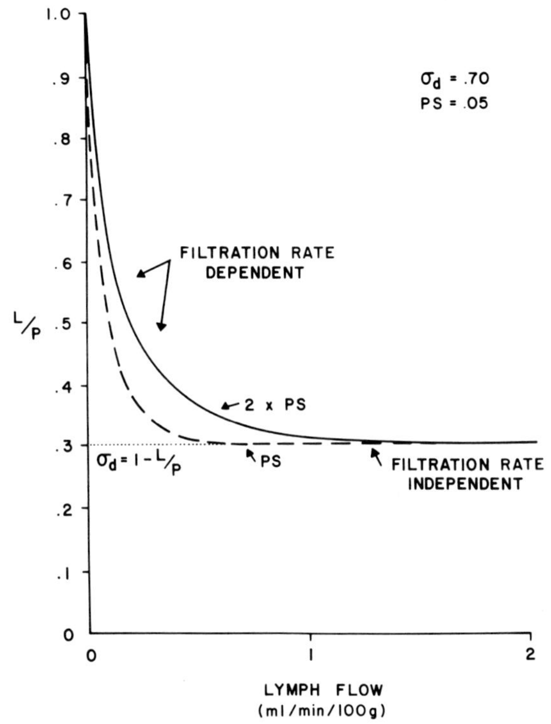

Fig. 2. Plot of protein concentration in lymph (L) relative to plasma (P) as a function of lymph flow. Note that even at higher surface areas that L/P approaches a constant at high lymph flows, i. e., is *filtration rate independent* (from [26], with permission).

occurs at a molecular radius of about 60 Å. Therefore, in our laboratory we used the experimental methods first applied in *Brigham*'s laboratory [4] to separate several endogenous proteins in lymph in order to evaluate σ_d for each individual plasma protein.

Figure 4 shows *Granger*'s [10] data for 9 different protein fractions as a function of molecular radius obtained at 4 different lymph flows. Note that C_L/C_P is smaller for larger proteins and the C_L/C_P for each protein fraction is smaller at each lymph flow. Although not shown on this graph, the C_L/C_P for each protein fraction also approached a constant at high lymph flow. How could we translate this information into a model which describes the endothelial barrier? *Renkin* [19, 20] had developed a means of representing macromolecular data by plotting $1-\sigma_d$ vs. solute radius for several endogenous plasma proteins and fitting the resulting data to two equivalent pores. Figure 5 shows a plot of *Renkin*'s analysis for $1-\sigma_d$ vs. molecular radius of seven different molecules across a three pore barrier having the molecular radii and number shown in the insert. The closed circles were first fit with a large pore fit (200 Å) using *Drake*'s equation, i. e., $\sigma = 16/3\,(a/r)^2 - 20/3\,(a/r)^3 + 7/3\,(a/r)^4$, where a is the solute radius and r the pore radius [7]. The points not falling on the 200 Å radius curve were analyzed in the following fashion: The 200 Å curve was subtracted from the points lying above in order to yield the open squares shown on

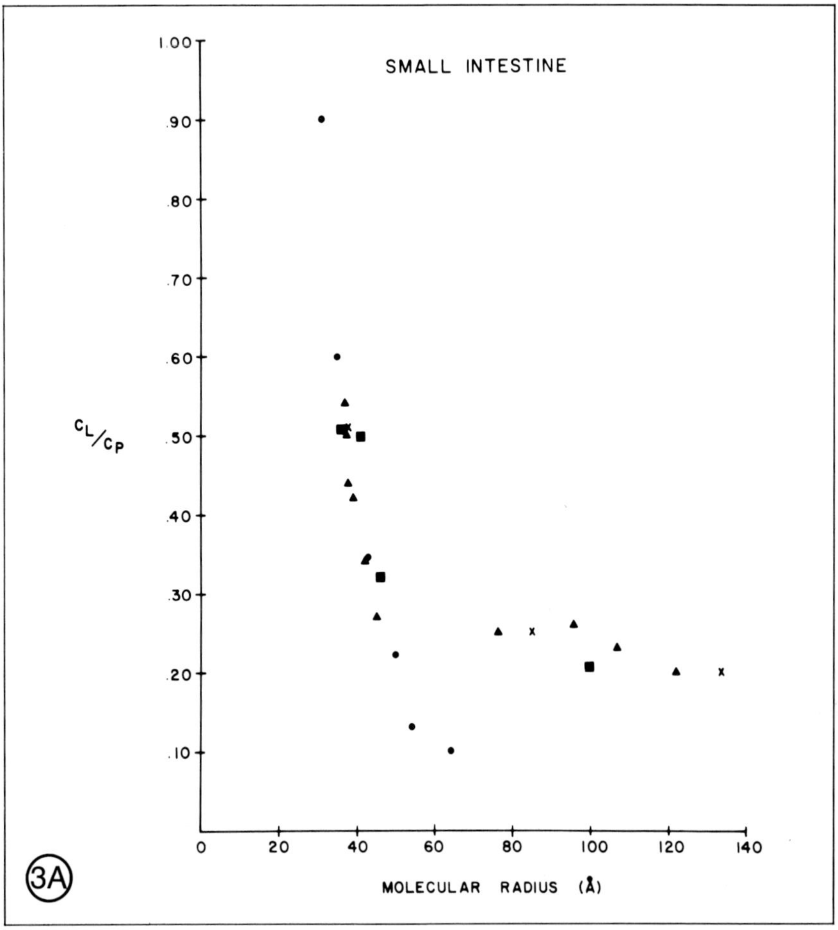

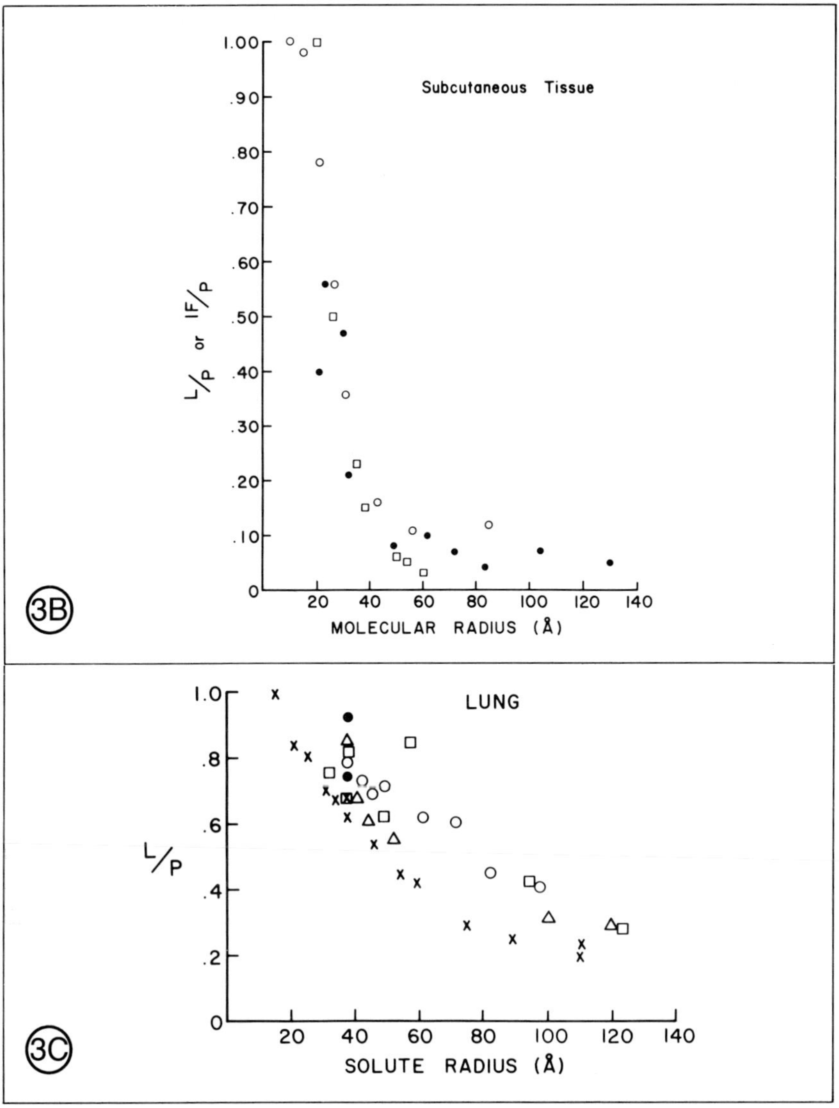

Fig. 3. A Plot of lymph to plasma ratio (C_L/C_P) of several different macromolecules as a function of molecular radius from intestinal lymph. *B* Plot of lymph to plasma ratios (L/P) of several different macromolecules in lymph and plasma as a function of molecular radius for lymph collected from subcutaneous tissue. IF refers to actual tissue samples of the macromolecule. *C* Plot of lymph to plasma ratios (L/P) of macromolecule in lung lymph. ○, △ and □ are endogenous protein fractions in dog and sheep lymph and x's are different sized PVPs (modified from [26]).

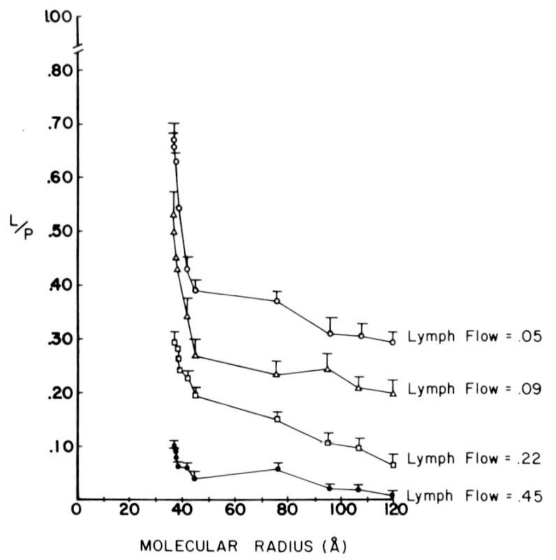

Fig. 4. Plot of lymph to plasma ratio (L/P) of 9 endogenous plasma proteins separated using gel electrophoresis from an intestinal preparation for which capillary pressure was elevated to produce 4 different lymph flow states. Note the smaller L/Ps for larger molecules and the dependency on lymph flow (from [25, 26]).

the curve. These points were then fit by another pore curve. This analysis predicts the different pore populations used to generate the data and the $1-\sigma_d$ intercept for each curve represents the percentage of the total volume flow occurring through each set of pores. Since the percentage of volume flow occurring through the small pores is 60% of the total membrane conductance and the large pore 35%, then 5% of the volume conductances resides in the 8 Å pores which is smaller than the smallest molecule used to generate the data. In addition, the number of small/large pores can be calculated as 1/149 using:

$$\frac{\text{number large pores}}{\text{number small pores}} = \frac{r^2_s}{r^2_1} \quad \frac{\text{large pore } (1-\sigma) \text{ intercept}}{\text{small pore } (1-\sigma) \text{ intercept}} \cdot \frac{r^2_s}{r^2_1}$$

Figure 6 A, B, C, and D show $1-\sigma_d$ as a function of solute radius for 9 different protein fractions obtained at 4 different flow rates (lymph flows). Note that the data can be fit by a set of large and small pores which appear to change at different filtration rates, and the calculated large to

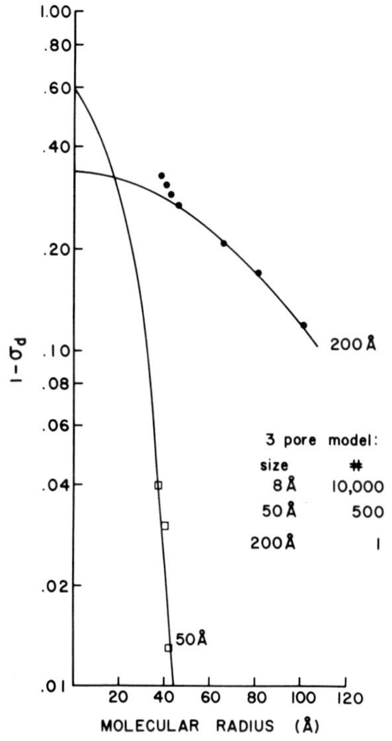

Fig. 5. Plot of one minus the reflection coefficient ($1-\sigma_d$) for 7 different sized macromolecules using *Renkin's* equation relating the volume conductance and σ_d. The pore radii and numbers are shown in the legends. The circles were fit with a 200 Å pore line. Then this 200 Å line was subtracted from the point lining above to produce the open squares which were then fit with a 50 Å pore. Note the excellent agreement between the pore sizes used to generate the data and the pore fits. The $1-\sigma_d$ intercept of the pore fit curves yield the percentage of the volume conductance (L_P) represented by this pore size. The 50 Å contains 60% of the membrane volume conductance, while the 200 Å pore represents 35% and the 8 Å pores represent 5% (from [26], with permission).

small pore numbers also change until from 1 : 1600 at low lymph flows to 1 : 6400. This explains why the linear equation (equation 1) fails to explain protein fluxes occurring across any heteroporous barriers. As the filtration increases, C_L/C_P for the different proteins will continue to change until the protein flux at each set of pores becomes filtration independent. At that C_L/C_P, further filtration will not alter the percentage of the flux occurring

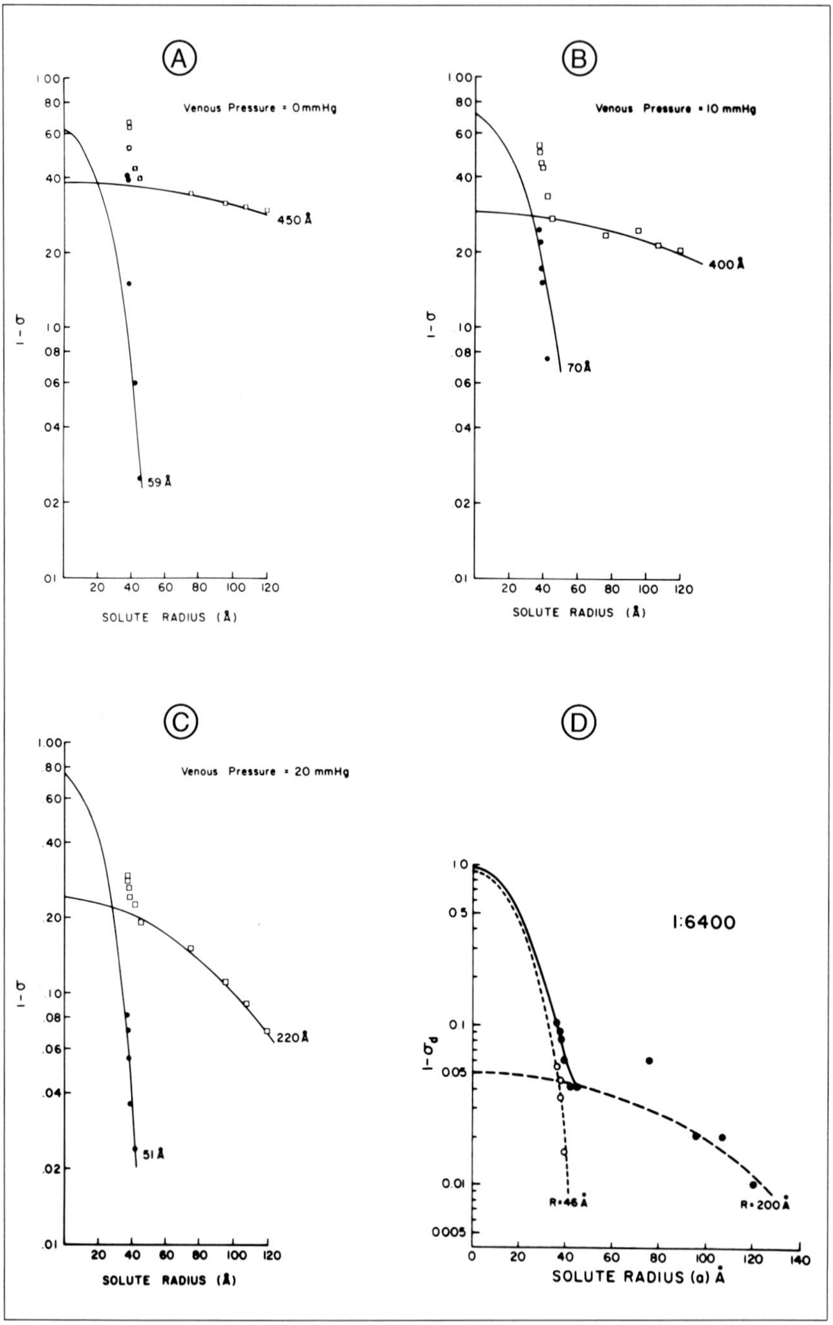
A
Venous Pressure = 0mmHg
450 Å
59 Å
1 - σ
SOLUTE RADIUS (Å)
B
Venous Pressure = 10 mmHg
400 Å
70 Å
1 - σ
SOLUTE RADIUS (Å)
C
Venous Pressure = 20 mmHg
220 Å
51 Å
1 - σ
SOLUTE RADIUS (Å)
D
1:6400
1-σd
R=46 Å
R=200 Å
SOLUTE RADIUS (a) Å

Table I. Predicted pore sizes and distribution in several capillary beds

Organ	Species	Small pore radius (Å)	Large pore radius (Å)	Fraction of hydraulic conductance through			Ratio of large-to-small pore	
				small pores	large pores	other	areas	numbers
Paw	Dog	47	195	0.82	0.13	0.05	1:141	1:2100
Lung	Dog	80	200	0.80	0.16	0.04	1:31	1:195
Skeletal muscle	Rat	67	220	0.65	0.018	0.33*	1:361	1:3610
Blood: CSF barrier	Man	70	180	0.86	0.10	0.04	1:52	1:345
Small intestine	Cat	46	200	0.90	0.05	0.05	1:340	1:6400
Stomach	Cat	47	250	0.75	0.23	0.02	1:92	1:2600
Colon	Dog	53	180	0.71	0.17	0.12	1:48	1:550
Liver	Cat	90	330	0.20	0.80	–	1:3.4	1:46

* Value calculated represents dilution caused by superfusion of muscle. Reprinted from [26]

through each set of pores. Then, and only then, a pore distribution describing the endothelial exchange barrier can be predicted.

Table I shows the results of using this type of analysis as applied to protein data obtained in several different vascular beds. Note, that although the vascular beds are somewhat different, most can be explained in terms of a 45–50 Å small pore population and a 200 Å large pore population.

Figure 7 shows another property when two different isomers of lactate dehydrogenase, a negative and a positive one, are collected in lymph. Note that molecular charge effects the concentration of plasma proteins in the lymph with more negative molecules showing higher C_L/C_Ps than positive macromolecules in both lung and the small intestinal lymph [15, 16, 29]. This is quite different from the glomerular barrier, which is a negative barrier [5]. Therefore, pore fits, as described in figures 5 and 6 in

Fig. 6. Pore fitting analysis applied to data collected from the small intestine at four different lymph flows (fig. 4). Note that the large pore size as well as relative number decreases as $C_L/C_P \rightarrow 1-\sigma_d$. Note that the $(1-\sigma_d)$ intercept (percentage of membrane volume conductance) decreases as $C_L/C_P \rightarrow 1-\sigma_d$; therefore, this analysis is only applicable when C_L/C_P is filtration independent and $\sigma_d = 1-C_L/C_P$ (with permission from [26]).

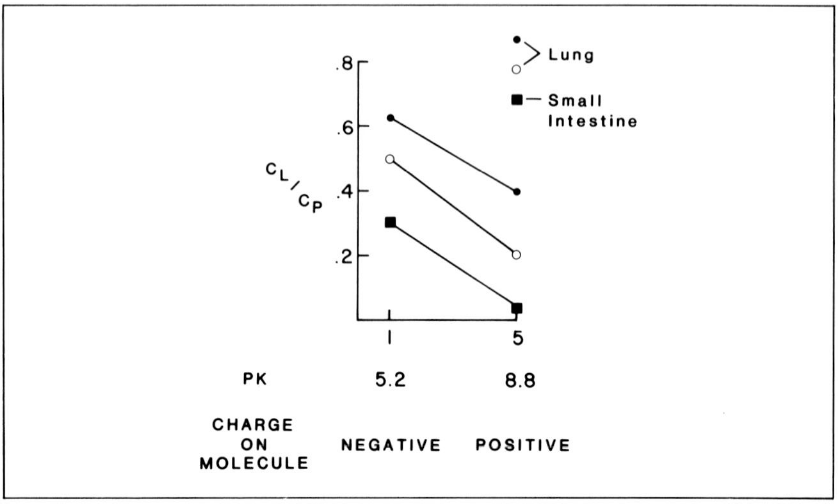

Fig. 7. Plot of C_L/C_P for two different isoenzymes of lactate dehydrogenase from intestine [15], and lung [16, 29]. Note that the more positive molecules have lower C_L/C_Ps indicating a positive-type barrier (from [25]).

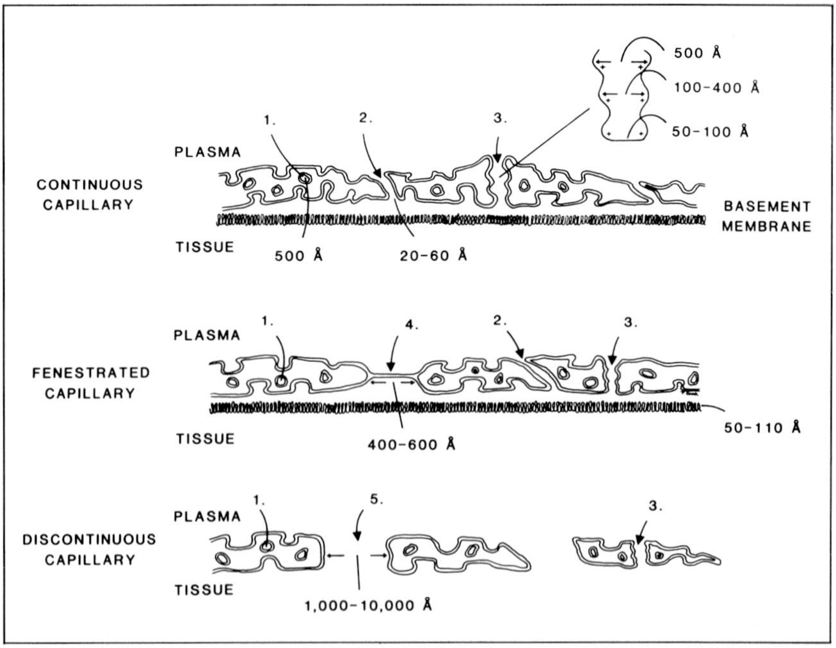

this paper, are related not only to molecular size and configuration but also are functions of molecular charge. This effect is currently under intense investigation since the pulmonary capillary endothelium appears to have a negative barrier located at its surface [23]. Dr. *Parker* [9], in our laboratory, feels that this apparent paradox may be the result of the positive macromolecules being delayed in attaining a steady-state until the negative tissue mucopolysaccharides are 'covered'. The possibility of a positive barrier is a puzzling finding and future work must provide the necessary information to unravel this strange phenomena, i. e., apparent capillary wall negativity – apparent capillary wall-lymphatic system positivity.

Structural Equivalents of 'Physiological Pores'

Figure 8 shows a schematic diagram of 3 different types of endothelium and the possible pathways associated with macromolecule transport. *1,* refers to pinocytotic vesicles; *2,* to endothelial junctions; *3,* to fused plasmalemmal vesicles; *4,* to fenestrae and *5* to endothelial gaps [25–28]. The most likely correlate for the physiological small and large pore systems are not apparent for the structures shown in figure 8, but the channels between endothelial cells in the venular end of the capillary system could be the structural counterpart of both the small and large pore systems. However, these structures should behave as negatively charged barriers and data from lymph appears to be best described as a positively charged barrier. A rather likely candidate for both the large and small pore system is shown as the insert in figure 8. The transendothelial channels formed by fused vesicles, form small pores if covered by a diaphragm and larger ones as indicated only by constriction sites. The dimensions of this structure are very similar to the 100 and 400 Å diameter pores predicted using lymphatic flux data. In addition, these structures may be

---

Fig. 8. Schematic representation of continuous, fenestrated and discontinuous capillary walls. The numbers 1–5 refer to plasmalemmal vesicles, endothelial junctions, transendothelial channels, fenestrations and openings in discontinuous capillary walls, respectively. The numbers refer to the diameters of the indicated structures, and a schematic transendothelial channel is shown in the top portion of the figure with its related structure and dimensions (from [25, 26]).

positively charged. Future work may provide data which produces better correlation between structural and physiological data, but the present data does not seem to fit into any logical scheme, with the exception of the fused transendothelial vesicles acting as both large and small pores.

Basic Assumptions which Must Be Met before Lymph Can Be Used to Assess Vascular Permeability to Macromolecules

Up to this point, we have indicated that lymph can be used to assess vascular permeability, but there are several experimental problems encountered when using lymph. Table II shows the requirements which must be experimentally met before lymph can be analyzed to yield information concerning the morphological characteristics of the endothelium of the microcirculation. For lymph to reflect tissue fluid requires that: first, the lymph must not be contaminated by sources other than the organ under study [6, 21]; secondly, the proteins in lymph must be at a steady-state and this may require several hours [26, 27]; thirdly, if the collection site is post-nodal, then the node can certainly add or subtract fluid and protein from the lymph [1, 2, 14]; fourthly, lymph fluid and protein cannot be exchanged across the larger lymphatic vessels [28]; and fifthly, there are no protein concentration gradients existing in the tissues [28].

A major assumption made when using lymph is that the major barrier to macromolecule movement resides at the endothelial-basement mem-

Table II. Basic assumptions made in analyzing lung lymph for assessment of vascular wall selectivity

1.: That the sampled lymphatic reflects lung tissue fluids. Requires that:
   (a) the lymph sampled is not contaminated by extrapulmonary sources;
   (b) the lymphatic proteins have sufficient time to equilibrate within the lung's tissue fluids during the experimental procedure;
   (c) nodes do not add or subtract fluid and protein from the collected lymph;
   (d) fluid and protein are not exchanged across collecting lymphatic vessel walls;
   (e) there are no gradients of protein concentrations in the interstitial spaces.

2.: That the major barrier to protein movement resides at the microvascular wall, not in the interstitium or at the lymphatic wall.

3.: That any charge effect of the vascular wall and interstitium on the movement of negative proteins is incorporated into the calculated permeability measurements (PS's) and vascular wall selectivities (σ's).

brane barrier, not the interstitium or lymphatic walls. And finally, when pore sizes are estimated they include charge, size and configuration, not just the latter two.

The usage of pre-nodal lymph and the requirement of obtaining a filtration independent C_L/C_P eliminates or minimizes the problems listed under 1 in table II, but the barrier to diffusion and molecular charge effects are not really known to any degree of certainty in most vascular beds. From data collected in the liver, it is highly unlikely that the interstitium is the limiting barrier and that the initial lymphatics can restrict the passage of macromolecules [26]. If the conditions listed in table II are met, then lymph proteins can be used to define physiological pore populations. However, this information may not be useful to describe protein fluxes occurring across a heteroporous barrier, with heterogeneous driving forces unless C_L/C_P is at a filtration independent state.

Summary

Macromolecule permeability across the capillary-interstitial-lymphatic barrier can be assessed by analyzing protein fluxes of endogenous plasma proteins in lymph when the ratio of the protein's concentration in lymph to its plasma concentration is filtration independent, i. e., the ratio remains constant even when lymph flow (capillary filtration) continues to increase.

When studies were conducted in several different capillary beds, the protein flux data (ignoring any charge effect) could be described using two sets of equivalent pores of 45–80 Å and 200–250 Å radii, which provides 80–95% and 5–10% of the total hydraulic conductance of the capillary wall, respectively. The amount of the total membrane conductance with equivalent pores less than the radius of albumin was < 5% in all organs studied. When relative negative and positive lactate dehydrogenase molecules (or dextrans) were studied, it appeared that the capillary-tissue-lymphatic barrier acts as a positive barrier. This finding is at variance with isotopic studies looking at transport between plasma and endothelial barriers. The finding regarding the charge distribution across the capillary-interstitial-lymphatic barrier indicate that molecular charge density across the entire barrier is either positive, the equilibration with tissues is a lengthy time process and/or that fused plasmalemmal vesicles provide the major route of protein transport between plasma and interstitium.

References

1 Adair, T. H.; Guyton, A. C.: Modification of lymph by lymph nodes. II. Effect of increased lymph node venous blood pressure. Am. J. Physiol. C *245:* H616–H622 (1983).

2 Adair, T. H.; Moffatt, D. S.; Paulsen, A. W.; Guyton, A. C.: Quantitation of changes in lymph protein concentration during lymph node transit. Am. J. Physiol. C *243:* H351–H359 (1982).

3 Brace, P. A.; Granger, D. N.; Taylor, A. E.: Analysis of lymphatic protein flux data. II. Effect of capillary heterogeneity in estimates of reflection-coefficients and PS products. Microvasc. Res. *14:* 215–226 (1977).

4 Brigham, K. L.; Owen, P. J.: Increased sheep lung vascular permeability caused by histamine. Circulation Res. *36:* 761–770 (1975).

5 Deen, W. M.; Satvat, B.; Jamieson, J. M.: Theoretical model for glomerular filtration of charged solutes. Am. J. Physiol. C *238:* F120–F139 (1980).

6 Drake, R. E.; Adair, T.; Traber, D.; Gabel, J.: Contamination of caudal mediastinal node efferent lymph in sheep. Am J. Physiol. C *241:* H354–H357 (1981).

7 Drake, R.; David, E.: A corrected equation for calculation of reflection coefficients. Microvasc. Res. *15:* 259 (1978).

8 Drinkcr, C. K.: Extravascular protein and the lymphatic system. Ann. N. Y. Acad. Sci. *46:* 807-821 (1946).

9 Gilchrist, S. A.; Parker, J. C.: Exclusion of charged molecules in the pulmonary interstitium. Microvasc. Res., in press (1985).

10 Granger, D. N.; Taylor, A. E.: Permeability of intestinal capillaries to endogenous macromolecules. Am. J. Physiol. C *238:* H457–H464 (1980).

11 Grotte, G.: Passage of dextran molecules across the blood-lymph barrier. Acta chir. scand. (suppl.) *211:* 1–84 (1956).

12 Kedem, O.; Katchalsky, A.: Thermodynamic analysis of the permeability of biological membranes to nonelectrolytes. Biochim. biophys. Acta *27:* 229–246 (1958).

13 Mayerson, H. S.; Wolfram, C. G.; Shirley H. H., Jr.; Wasserman, K.: Regional differences in capillary permeability. Am J. Physiol. *198:* 155–160 (1960).

14 Maron, M. B.: Modification of lymph during passage through the lymph node: effect of histamine. Am. J. Physiol. C *245:* H553–H559 (1983).

15 McElearney, P. M.; Granger, D. N.: Intestinal wall as a charge-selective filter. Physiologist, Wash. *22:* 85 (1975).

16 Parker, R. E.; Richardson, D.; Granger, D.; Roselli, R.; Harris, T.; Brigham, K.: Charge permselectivity of the lung blood-lymph barrier in sheep. Fed. Proc. *40:* 449 (1981).

17 Patlak, C. S.; Goldstein, D. A.; Hofman, J. F.: The flow of solute and solvent across a two membrane system. J. theor. Biol. *5:* 425–442 (1963).

18 Perry, M. A.; Benoit, J. N.; Kvietys, P. R.; Granger, D. N.: Restricted transport of cationic macromolecules across intestinal capillaries. Am. J. Physiol. C *245:* G568–G572 (1983).

19 Renkin, E. M: Transport of proteins by diffusion, bulk flow and vesicular mechanism. Physiologist, Wash. *24:* 57–71 (1980).

20 Renkin, E. M.; Watson, P. D.; Sloop, C. H.; Joyner, W. L.; Curry, F. E.: Transport pathways for fluid and large molecules in microvascular endothelium of the dog's paw. Microvasc. Res. *14:* 205–214 (1977).

21 Roos, P. J.; Weiner-Kronish, J. P.; Albertine, K. H.; Staub, N. C.: Removal of abdominal sources of caudal mediastinal node lymph in anesthetized sheep. J. appl. Physiol. *55:* 996–1001 (1983).

22 Rutili, G.; Granger, D. N.; Parker, J. C.; Mortillaro, N. A.; Taylor, A. E.: Analysis of lymphatic protein data. IV. Comparison of the different methods used to estimate reflection coefficients and permeability surface area products. Microvasc. Res. *23:* 347–360 (1982).
23 Simionescu, N.; Simionescu, M.; Palade, G. E.: Differentiated microdomains on the luminal surface of the capillary endothelium. I. Preferential distribution of anionic sites. J. Cell Biol. *90:* 606–613 (1981).
24 Taylor, A. E.; Granger, D. N.; Brace, R. A.: Analysis of lymphatic protein flux. I. Estimation of the reflection coefficient and permeability surface area products for total plasma proteins. Microvasc. Res. *13:* 297–313 (1977).
25 Taylor, A. E.; Granger, D. N.: Equivalent pore modeling: Vesicles and channels. Fed. Proc. *42:* 2440–2445 (1983).
26 Taylor, A. E.; Granger, D. N.: Exchange of macromolecules across the circulation; in Renkin, Michel (eds.), Handbook of Physiology, Sect. 2, The Cardiovascular System, vol. IV, The Microcirculation, pp. 467–520 (American Physiological Society, Bethesda, 1984).
27 Taylor, A. E.; Parker, J. C.: The pulmonary interstitial spaces and lymphatics; in Fishman, Fisher (eds.), Handbook of Physiology, Respiration, vol. IV, pp. 167–320 (American Physiological Society, Bethesda, 1984).
28 Taylor, A. E.; Townsley, M. I.; Korthuis, R. J.: Macromolecule transport across the pulmonary microvascular walls. Exp. Lung Res., in press (1985).
29 Weaver; L. J.; Gleisner, J.; Winn, R.; Mansfield, E.; Stothert, J.; Hildebrandt, J.: Electrical potential ($\Delta\Psi$) and differences in lymph-plasma (L/P) ratios of molecules of similar size but differing charge. Fed. Proc. *41:* 1246 (1982).

A. E. Taylor, PhD, Department of Physiology, College of Medicine, University of South Alabama, Mobile, AL 36688 (USA)

Prog. appl. Microcirc., vol. 9, pp. 116–117 (Karger, Basel 1985)

Discussion of the Presentations: *O'Morchoe, Taylor*

CRONE: I would like to come back to the vesicular transport theory for macromolecules. How can we explain a reflection coefficient of 0.8–0.9 according to the classical vesicular transport hypothesis? One would expect to have a reflection coefficient of 1.0, because a vesicle has a cell membrane and it takes the plasma droplet and transports it through. That should give a reflection coefficient of 1.0, in my vocabulary, but I may be wrong.

TAYLOR: It looks to me like you could get quite a large bulk of things into a vesicle. You can go up to fairly large proteins, and ferry them across, but I don't think you ferry.

CRONE: No, but let us assume that for the sake of the argument. What should be the reflection coefficient if that is the way proteins are transported?

TAYLOR: It would look like diffusion, but as we analyze lymph we wouldn't know what it meant. It would just be some molecules appearing in the lymph.

CRONE: That is not a satisfactory answer.

TAYLOR: I think it is.

MICHEL: Can I try to answer this? I agree with Dr. CRONE. The reflection coefficient, if you had classical vesicular transport, would appear in a membrane to be very, very close to one. There is a small correction, which is due to the volume flux of the protein. The physiological evidence which suggests that there might be a vesicular transport is the indirect evidence that there exists a component of macromolecular permeability which is independent of convective flow through the capillary wall. That is the only physiological evidence for it.

CRONE: I quite agree with you, but what I wanted to stress is the fact, that the reflection coefficient is clearly, as found by everybody, below one and that tells us that there is also a channel where water and protein come in together.

TAYLOR: Oh yes, I know that. I was thinking, that if you had vesicles only, you would be dumping some protein into the interstitium, which would wind up in lymph.

CRONE: All I want is to remind us about some basic facts, which we have to explain one way or another. The reflection coefficient is always less than one, and that cannot be explained according to the 'classical' concept of *Palade*.

TAYLOR: I still cannot say that one wouldn't have proteins going across, if they go across.

CRONE: Of course they would go, but they would go across with a reflection coefficient of one.

TAYLOR: Perhaps the vesicles are selective. It always appeared to me like taking some proteins from here and transferring them over there, and we have always said that that acted like diffusion. If that is what you're saying, I agree.

PIETRA: I'm a little concerned by the fact that you seem to put the pore only in the endothelium. Are you excluding completely the influence of basement membrane, particularly for the data on the charged molecules?

TAYLOR: We really thought that we were looking at the basement membrane, but that again is purely speculation. In fact I think that we said in our Handbook article, it may be the basement membrane, provided it is positively charged.

END OF DISCUSSION

Prog. appl. Microcirc., vol. 9, pp. 118–134 (Karger, Basel 1985)

Bulk Flow of Humors of the Eye and Brain through Vacuolar Transendothelial Channels*

R. C. Tripathi, B. J. Tripathi

Eye Research Laboratories, University of Chicago, Chicago, Ill., USA

Introduction

The close analogy between the aqueous humor of the eye and the cerebrospinal fluid (CSF) of the brain has been scrutinized extensively by *Davson* [4–6]. Both of these clear, colorless fluids perform important hydromechanical functions while maintaining a steady state intraocular and intracranial pressure. The aqueous humor, in conjunction with the fibrous tunics of the eye, provides stability to the ocular dimensions and to the internal structures of the eye in the performance of its visual function. Similarly, the CSF supports the weight of the brain and acts as a hydraulic shock absorber against external mechanical forces. Both fluids carry away metabolic wastes and toxic metabolites, supply nutrients, distribute neurohormonal agents, and provide a constant environment for the normal functioning of the tissues that they bathe.

The hydromechanical and metabolic functions of aqueous humor and CSF call for their continuous formation and drainage: in man, approximately 3 ml of aqueous humor and 500 ml of CSF are formed and drained away daily. It is now generally recognized that aqueous humor escapes from the anterior chamber of the eye into the canal of Schlemm (fig. 1A) and cerebrospinal fluid escapes from the subarachnoid space of the brain into the dural sinuses (fig. 1B) by bulk flow; i. e., all matter in these fluids, whether present naturally or introduced experimentally, leaves by mass transfer at the same rate.

* It is our privilege to dedicate this paper to our esteemed friend and mentor, Professor *Hugh Davson,* D.Sc., to commemorate his 75th birthday.

The history of investigations into the outflow mechanisms of both fluids spans well over a century. With a few notable exceptions, investigators of the eye and brain have worked independently of each other. It is remarkable, however, that the mechanisms proposed for the outflow of these two fluids and the research approaches to them are basically similar. The proposed mechanisms for passage across the endothelial barrier may be summarized as one, or a combination, of the following: diffusion, osmosis, intercellular leakage, active transport, and passage through endothelium-lined channels. None of these mechanisms, however, has provided a satisfactory explanation for the steady state pressure, the bulk flow, and the rate of outflow across the cellular barrier of the endothelial

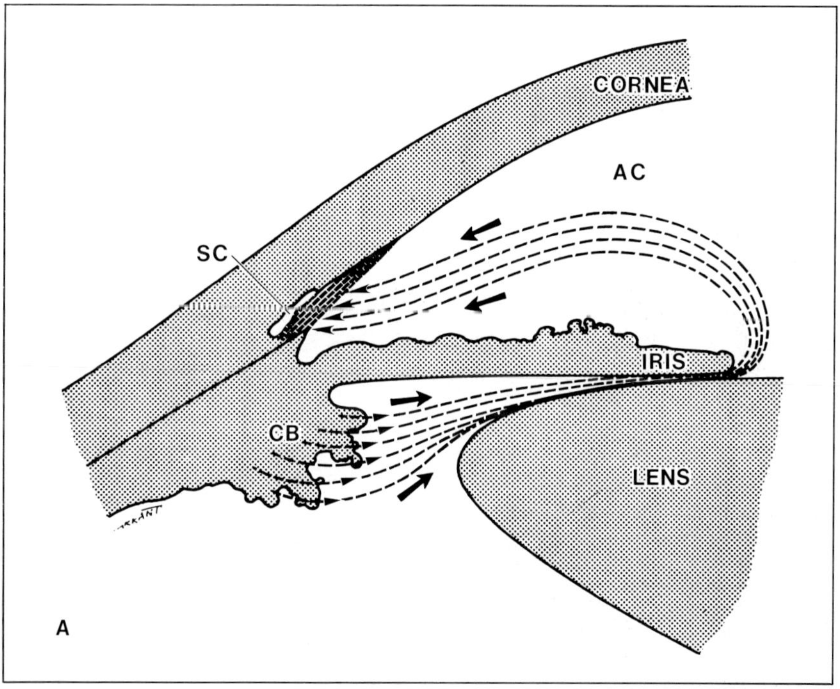

Fig. 1A. Diagrammatic representation of the circulatory pathway of aqueous humor in the primate eye. The fluid is formed in the posterior chamber by the ciliary body (CB) and enters into the anterior chamber (AC) through the pupil. The bulk outflow of aqueous humor takes place into the lumen of Schlemm's canal (SC) by traversing its endothelial barrier. From Schlemm's canal, the aqueous humor is drained away by luminal flow into the episcleral venous system and finally into the systemic circulation.

lining of Schlemm's canal in the eye and across that of the arachnoid villi/granulations in the brain. It is for this reason that we investigated the morphologic and physiologic bases governing the bulk flow of these fluids and introduced the concept of cyclically formed vacuolar transcellular channels. In this presentation, we will briefly examine the similarity of our proposed system to transcellular channels existing in other biological systems.

Material and Methods

For this series of investigations, normal eyes from a wide variety of vertebrate species (e.g., man; non-human primates; sub-primate mammals including rabbit, dog, cat, rat, ox, horse, sheep, camel, zebra, kangaroo, duck-billed platypus; birds; reptiles; amphibia; as well

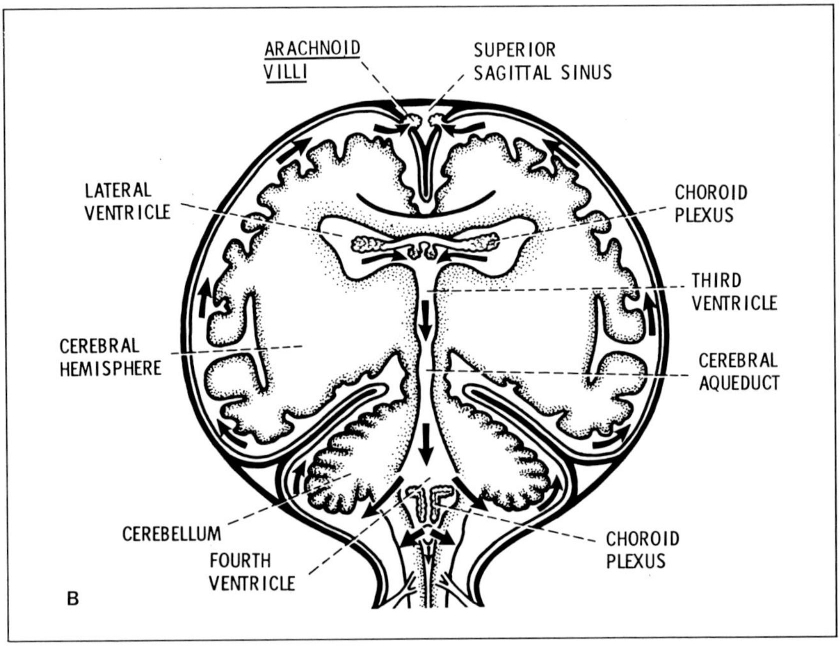

Fig. 1B. Diagrammatic representation of the circulatory pathway of CSF in the primate central nervous system. The fluid is formed in the lateral and fourth cerebral ventricles by the choroidal plexuses and escapes into the subarachnoid space through the foramina of Magendie and Luschka, which are located at the base of the brain. CSF is drained away by bulk flow across the endothelial barrier of arachnoid villi/granulations that herniate into the dural venous sinuses.

as teleost and cartilaginous fish) were studied by light microscopy and by transmission and scanning electron microscopy. The leptomeninges of the brain were studied from a limited number of mammalian species. Details of the methods employed have been documented elsewhere [16, 18, 20]. Briefly, the tissues were fixed at normal intraocular and intracisternal pressure with 3% buffered isotonic glutaraldehyde or a glutaraldehyde/paraformaldehyde mixture according to one of the following protocols:

(1) Intravitally by intracardiac or intracarotid perfusion with a sustained pressure perfusion technique;

(2) by intracameral or intracisternal perfusion fixation at a controlled pressure;

(3) by immersion fixation of freshly and rapidly excised tissue.

Block staining was performed for histochemical reaction or contrast enhancement. Aldehyde-fixed tissues were routinely postfixed in 1% buffered osmium tetroxide. Appropriate tissue blocks were dehydrated in ethanol, embedded in epoxy-resin for semi-thin and ultrathin sections, and, after appropriate staining reactions, examined by light microscopy and transmission electron microscopy, respectively. For scanning electron microscopy, tissue blocks were dehydrated in ethanol and acetone or amyl acetate, critical point dried, and coated with gold palladium.

To trace the outflow pathway of aqueous humor and CSF, we introduced markers such as colloidally suspended Thorotrast, ferritin serum solution, colloidal gold, horseradish peroxidase, lanthanum red, latex spheres of various sizes, or autogenous whole blood into the anterior chamber of the eye and into the cisterna magna of the brain at controlled pressures. After varying time intervals, the tissues were fixed according to one of the protocols outlined above. To evaluate the effect of pressure on the lining endothelial cells, we carried out perfusion experiments at graded levels of intracameral and intracisternal pressures (0 mm Hg to 40 mm Hg) for 10 to 30 min, and tissues were fixed at the same pressure for light and electron microscopic studies.

Results

Gross morphologic differences were noted in the organization of the angular region of the eye in various species and the leptomeninges of the brain [18–20]. However, within species, the endothelial linings of the trabecular wall of the canal of Schlemm in the eye and of the arachnoid villi and granulations in the brain showed remarkable similarities. Both linings consisted of a single layer of elongated and flattened cells, which measured about 80 to 120 μm in length, 4 to 12 μm in width, and 0.5 to 8 μm in thickness, the latter measurement being taken at the location of the nucleus and/or macrovacuolar structures. A thin, discontinuous basement membrane adhered to the basal aspect of the cells. Adjacent cell borders often overlapped and were joined by occluding zonules that occupied only a small area of the cell surface [14, 20]. The cells contained the usual intracellular organelles, such as a centrally located oblong nucleus, moder-

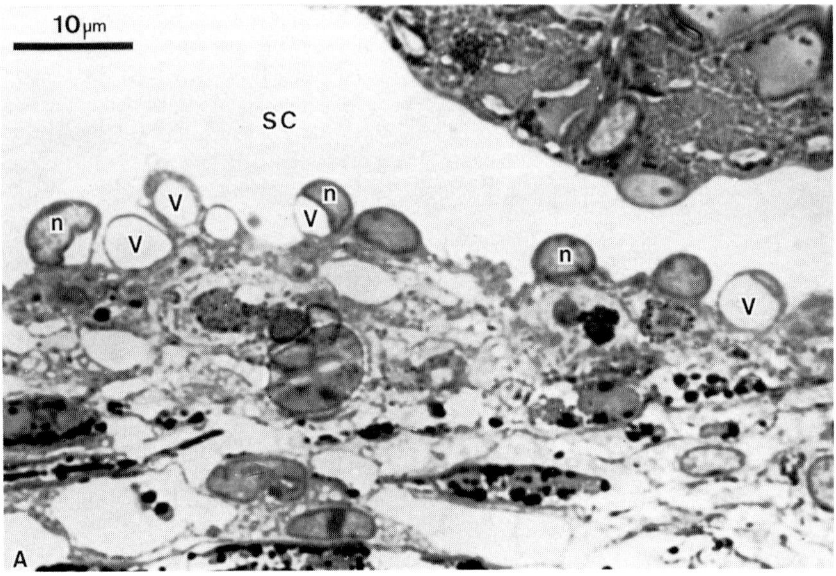

Fig. 2A. A portion of Schlemm's canal (SC) in meridional section. In this normotensive monkey eye, the trabecular wall is lined by a single layer of endothelial cells characterized by bulging nuclei (n) and macrovacuolar configurations (V). Epoxy-resin-embedded tissue. Photomicrograph × 1,600.

ate numbers of small mitochondria, as well as endoplasmic reticulum, Golgi apparatus, membrane-bound dense bodies, multivesicular bodies, centrosomes, pinocytotic vesicles, glycogen, and ribonucleic acid granules. The cytoskeletal system of the cells included numerous intermediate filaments (8–10 nm in diameter), together with some actin filaments (5–7 nm in diameter) and microtubules (ca. 10 nm in diameter).

In the normotensive state of the eye and subarachnoid space, the striking feature of the lining endothelial cells was the presence of giant vacuolar configurations (fig. 2A). All vacuoles were unit-membrane-bound, and their limiting membrane was smooth and of the same thickness as the cell plasmalemma. The vacuoles were generally electron-optically empty, although some contained a flocculent material similar to the subendothelial basement membrane and ground substance. They were generally globular in shape, bulging into the lumen of Schlemm's canal or into the dural sinus. The largest vacuole measured up to 4 μm × 7 μm × 25 μm, the long axis being parallel to that of the endothelial cells. Vacuolar configurations located centrally in the cell displaced the nucleus, giving it a crescent shape (figs. 2A and 2B). Some of the vacuolar configurations were multilocular or followed a sinuous course through the cell.

Random sections through vacuolar configurations revealed the following profiles:

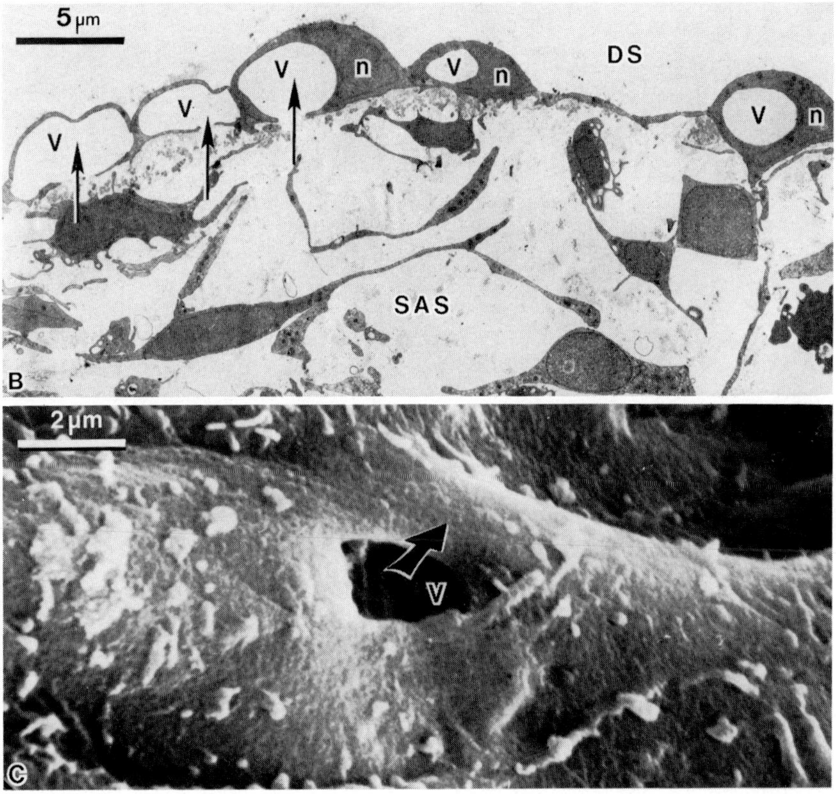

Fig. 2B. Survey electron micrograph of a portion of arachnoid villus in the monkey showing its continuous endothelial lining, many cells of which contain macrovacuolar structures (V) bulging into the dural sinus (DS). Arrows indicate the communication of vacuolar structures with the underlying extracellular spaces of the subarachnoid system (SAS). n = Nuclei of endothelial lining. Micrograph 2,800 ×.

Fig. 2C. Scanning electron micrograph of the endothelium lining the arachnoid villus, seen from the dural sinus aspect. One of the giant vacuolar configurations (V) shows a natural opening (arrow) into the dural sinus. Micrograph 6,900 ×.

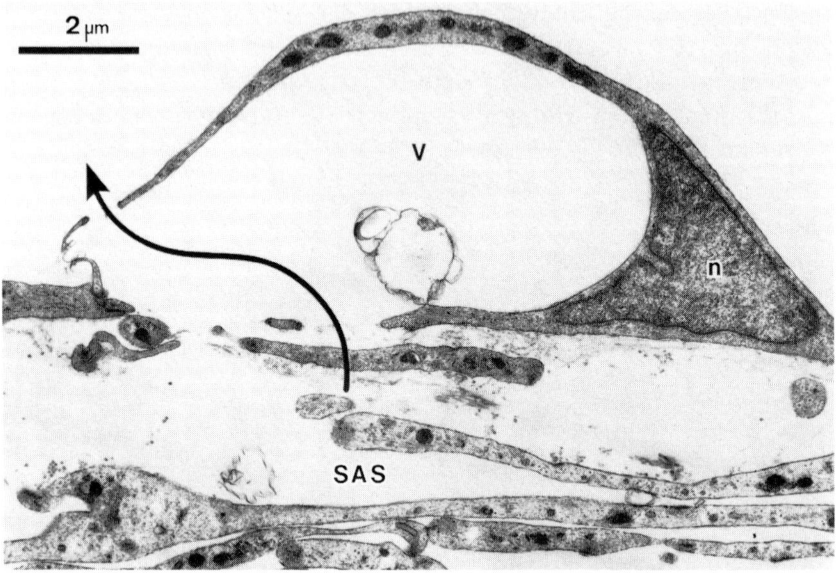

Fig. 3. Electron micrograph of a macrovacuolar configuration in a lining cell of the arachnoid villus. In this section, the basal and apical openings of the macrovacuole (V) are shown by an arrow representing unidirectional flow of CSF. n = Nucleus displaced to one side of the endothelial cell to accommodate the macrovacuole; SAS = subarachnoid space. Micrograph 7,800 ×.

(1) Vacuoles in communication with the subendothelial extracellular space through the basal aspect of the cell surface, the openings measuring up to 4 μm (fig. 2B);

(2) vacuoles appearing to be entirely within a single endothelial cell (fig. 2B) ;

(3) vacuoles communicating with the lumen of Schlemm's canal or of the dural sinus through the apical aspect of the cell surface, which measured up to 2.5 μm (fig. 2C); and

(4) vacuoles having communication with both the basal and apical aspects of the cell surface, thus forming a transendothelial channel (fig. 3).

Analysis of serial sections revealed that the various profiles were related to the plane of the section through the vacuolar configurations. A statistical survey showed that, normally at a given time, only about 2% of all vacuoles constituted transcellular channels; the majority of the vacuoles had a ballooned profile with a narrow basal opening and, in fact,

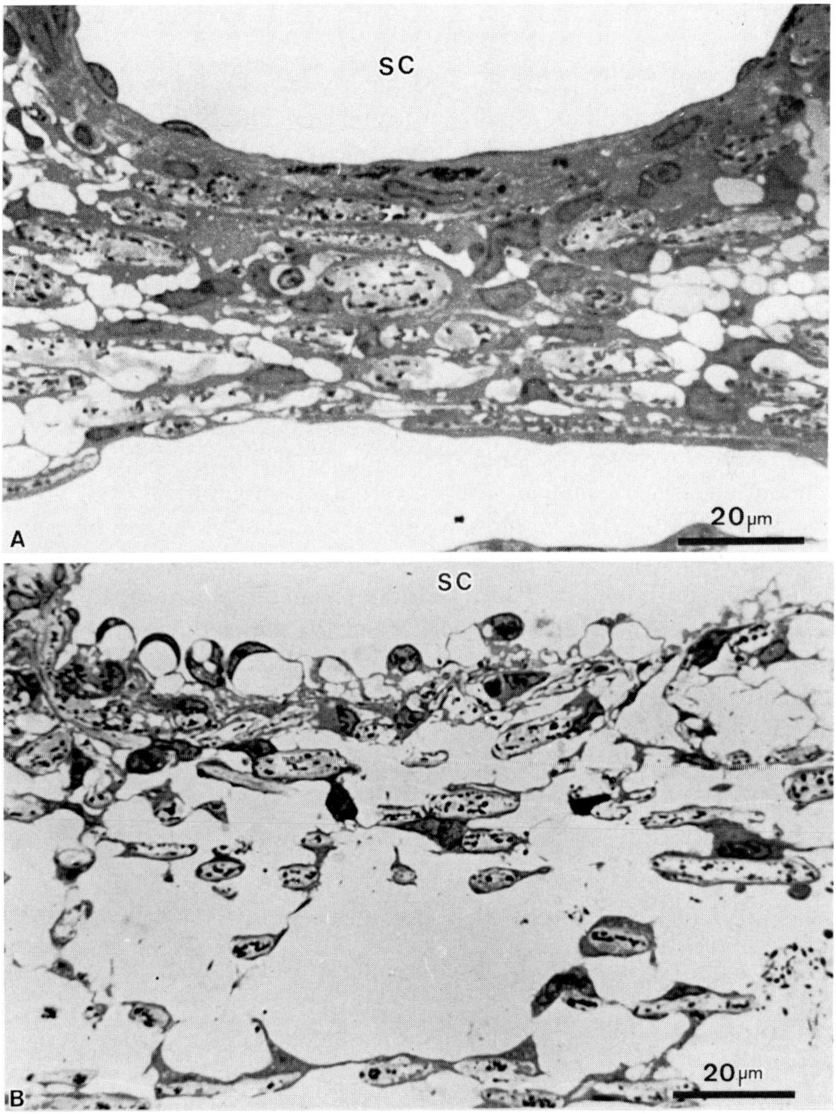

Fig. 4. Profiles of the trabecular wall of Schlemm's canal and underlying trabecular meshwork. Following hypotony, vacuolar configurations in the endothelial lining of Schlemm's canal (SC) disappear and the subendothelial tissue becomes compact, as seen in figure 4A. Experimentally elevated intraocular pressure increases the number and size of macrovacuolar configurations and causes widening of subendothelial tissue, as seen in figure 4B. Epoxy-resin embedded tissue. Photomicrographs 800 ×.

represented an extension of the extracellular space as a diverticulum into a deformed cell.

Experimental studies with tracer materials revealed that the vacuolar configurations were filled rapidly through the opening that communicated with the basal extracellular space. The vacuolar configurations which also had an opening on the apical surface of the cell showed leakage of tracer material into the lumen of Schlemm's canal or of the dural sinus. Unlike the macrovacuolar configurations, the micropinocytotic vesicles rarely contained the tracer material within the approximately 20 min duration of the experiments; particles 10 nm or larger were not seen traversing the intercellular junctions. When whole blood was used as a tracer, intact blood cells, including erythrocytes, could be identified in transit, indicating biopedesis through the vacuolar configurations. Some leukocytic cells were seen traversing the flat part of individual lining endothelial cells without apparent formation of macrovacuolar configurations [20, 22].

When the pressure within the anterior chamber of the eye or in the subarachnoid space of the brain was lowered to 0 mm Hg, the vacuolar configurations in the endothelial cells disappeared rapidly, usually within a few minutes. The endothelial cells assumed a thin and flattened profile and the subendothelial connective tissue became compact (fig. 4A). An increase in intraocular or subarachnoid pressure produced the opposite effect: the number and size of the vacuolar configurations increased, and the subendothelial tissue region became distended with the enlargement of the extracellular spaces (fig. 4B).

Discussion

The normal presence of macrovacuoles in the endothelial lining of Schlemm's canal is now recognized by many investigators [cf. 2, 6, 11, 20, 22]. Based on our morphologic and experimental studies, we postulate that the giant vacuolar configurations in the endothelial cells lining Schlemm's canal in the eye and in the arachnoid villi in the brain are intimately involved with the bulk outflow of aqueous humor and CSF, respectively. The results of our experiments suggest that the vacuolar configurations are not static structures, but dynamic entities which, through a cyclical sequence of events, form a system of transcellular pathways to allow outflow of aqueous humor and CSF (fig. 5).

We believe that the vacuolar configuration begins to develop from an

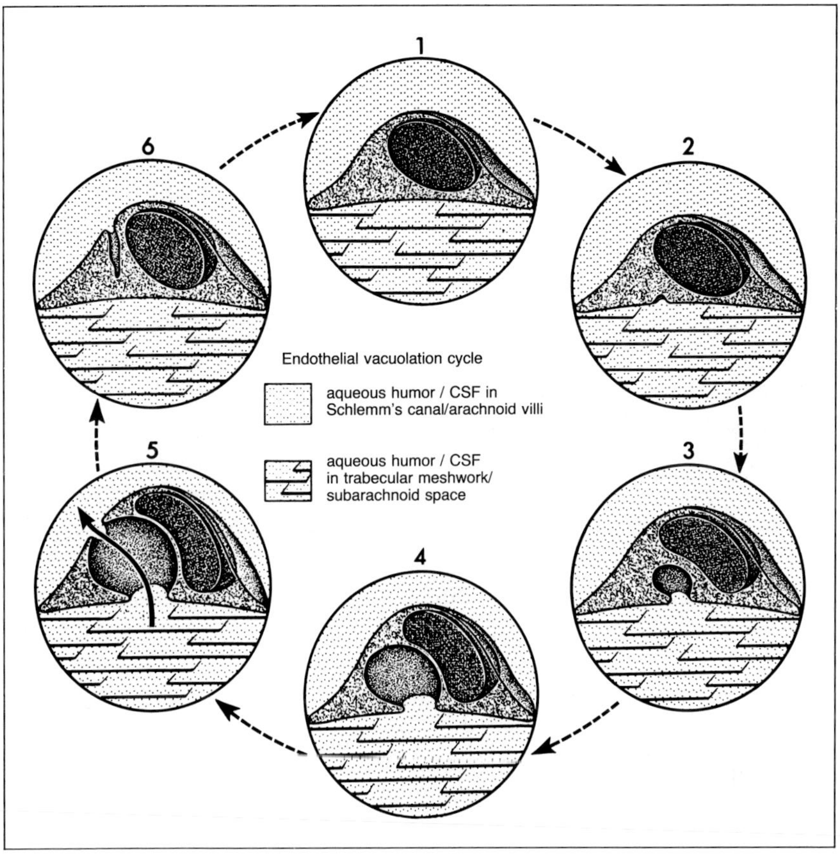

Fig. 5. Schematic representation of cyclical sequence of events in the formation of a dynamic system of transient transcellular channels. A transcellular channel is formed through gradual invagination of the plasma membrane on the basal cell surface, probably in response to transendothelial hydrostatic pressure through a pressure-sensitive receptor-mediated mechanism (stages 2–4). Fusion of basal and apical cell plasmalemma creates a transcellular channel that temporarily connects the extracellular space on the basal aspect of the cell to its luminal aspect. The bulk flow of aqueous humor and CSF occurs down a pressure gradient through such channels (stage 5). A reduction in the transendothelial pressure gradient leads to regression of vacuolization (stages 6 and 1). (Adapted from *Tripathi* [20]).

invagination or indentation in the basal cell membrane as a macroendocytotic pit. This probably occurs in response to the hydrostatic pressure at selective, pressure-sensitive sites. The invaginations are usually located in the central region of the basal aspect of the lining cells. The indentation expands gradually to form a larger balloon-shaped invagination, and the basal plasmalemma eventually comes in contact with the inner aspect of the apical cell membrane. A fusion of the two membranes results in the formation of a vacuolar transendothelial channel, i. e., the cell is completely traversed by a membrane-lined channel, which temporarily connects the extracellular space on the basal aspect of the cell to the lumen of Schlemm's canal or of the dural sinus (fig. 5, stage 5). This through-and-through communication from the basal to the apical aspect of the cell allows the bulk flow of aqueous humor or CSF down a pressure gradient. After a certain interval, as the pressure on the basal aspect becomes lower, the recoil property of the cell, which is probably imparted by cytoskeleton-plasma membrane interactions, helps to seal the basal opening, and occlusion of the apical opening follows; thus, vacuolization is reversed. A profile of the endothelial cells lining Schlemm's canal and of the vacuolation process forming transcellular channels is shown schematically in figure 6.

Statistical analysis reveals that the vacuolar transendothelial channels are heterogeneous in size, and that they occupy only a short time span, about one-fiftieth of the total life cycle of the vacuoles [3]. Normally, the total number and the size of transcellular channels are, however, sufficient to maintain the observed rate of flow of aqueous humor and CSF, thus regulating the steady state of intraocular and intracranial pressure. That these channels act as one-way valves, i. e., allow the flow of fluid from the basal to the apical aspect of the cells far more easily than vice versa, is suggested by their morphologic configuration, including their larger basal opening compared with the apical opening, the latter being located tangentially at the convex surface of the vacuolar configuration and not directly opposite the basal opening. The transcellular channels often take a sinuous course through the cell. Our experimental evidence suggests that, with reversed pressure, these channels, in conjunction with the contractile property of the cell, act as one-way self-sealing valves.

Our experimental studies demonstrated that the vacuolar configurations are uniquely pressure-sensitive, normally operating within a pressure range of only a few mm Hg, and that the number and location of macrovacuoles are influenced by the transendothelial hydrostatic pressure

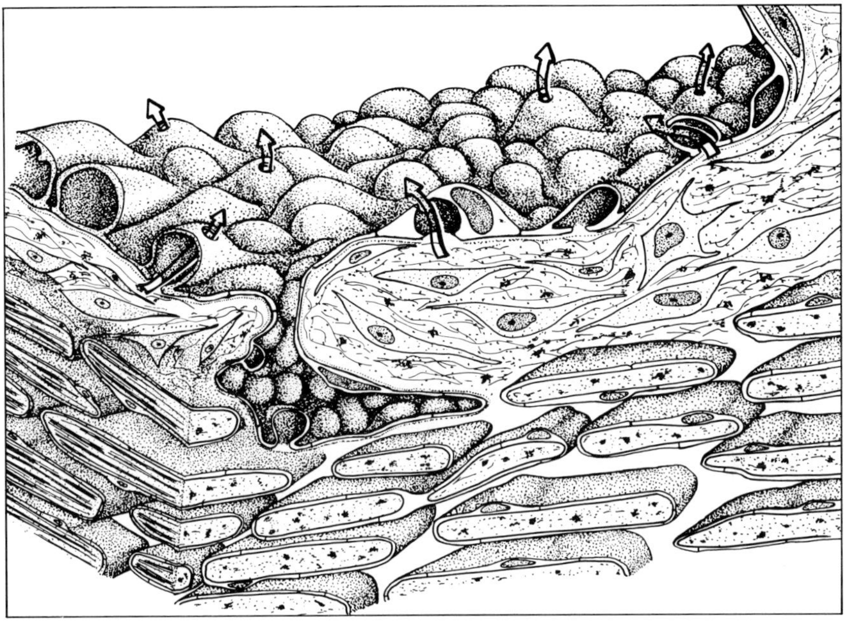

Fig. 6. Schematic representation of endothelial lining of Schlemm's canal, depicting the macrovacuolar configurations that provide a pathway for the bulk outflow of aqueous humor (arrows).

gradient in a given region of the canal of Schlemm and of the arachnoid villi. We have further concluded that, in order to preserve the true size, number, and configuration of the vacuolar structures, the endothelial cells lining Schlemm's canal and the arachnoid villi must be fixed for microscopic studies at the pressure preexisting in the anterior chamber of the eye and in the subarachnoid space of the brain. Failure to do so will result in erroneous conclusions as to the nature of the macrovacuoles.

In postulating our theory of a cyclical sequence of events in the genesis of vacuolar configurations, we have considered several alternatives; these include the possibility of:

(1) permanently opened transcellular channels,

(2) vacuoles originating in the cell cytoplasm (similar to the contractile vacuole of the amoeba) which eventually open on both the apical and basal aspect of the cell, and

(3) macropinocytotic transport [3, 16, 19, 20].

On physiologic and morphologic grounds, however, none of these mechanisms can account for the bulk outflow of fluid, for the linearity of the pressure/flow relationship, or for the maintenance of steady state hydrodynamics in the eye and brain [2, 20].

We have given consideration to various factors, such as physical and chemical properties of the aqueous humor and CSF, neuronal and hormonal agents, cellular metabolism, as well as homeostasis, which may control the vacuolation process in the eye and brain. Pressure-dependent phenomena are widespread among members of the animal kingdom, but the mechanism by which organisms and cells perceive the pressure stimulus remains an enigma. A cellular response to pressure could be triggered by one factor or a combination of several factors, e. g., changes in cell volume, changes in hydration and mobility of certain ions associated with an alteration in the trans-membrane potential, stimulation of enzyme(s), or changes in cellular viscosity [cf. 13]. The pressure sensitivity of cells may also be due to an electrode effect arising from compression of hydrogen that is produced electrolytically on the outer surface [9]. Conceivably, in the case of the eye and of the brain, the plasma membrane of the endothelial cells is specially endowed with a receptor for pressure sensitivity. This may be in the form of a protein inserted in the membrane structure, and it may confer a property of deformability somewhat similar to that of the red cell membrane [10].

Passage of fluid or foreign material through the body of a single cell, i. e., transcellular passage, is not confined to the endothelial cells in the eye and brain. In fact, it appears to be a widespread and fundamental phenomenon serving a number of purposes. Sponges represent an ancient group of sessile animals in which flow of environmental water through the body of the sponge is created in order for it to obtain nutrients. The water passes through the cell cytoplasm of special pore cells or 'porocytes'. In some species, the flow of water is regulated by contractile cells located around the porocytes. Recently, evidence has been presented for one-way valves in the water-flow system of sponges [23], which provides a further analogy with the transendothelial channels that permit the bulk outflow of aqueous humor and CSF. However, the fundamental difference between the transcellular passage of fluid in sponges and in the endothelial cells of the eye and brain is that the former represents the function of a permanent structure, whereas in the latter, temporary vacuolar channels are formed through a cyclical sequence of events [16, 18–20].

In some capillary endothelial cells, a transcellular migration of material is known to occur through chains of vesicles that form patent microvesicular transendothelial tubules and connect temporarily the basal and apical endothelial cell surfaces [12, 15]. Low-molecular-weight tracers can traverse the cell by this mechanism. However, compared with the macrovacuolar configurations several μm in size that normally form transendothelial channels in the lining of Schlemm's canal and of arachnoid villi, the microvesicular transendothelial tubules are extremely small (diameter ca. 11 nm) and serve a rather limited purpose.

The selective passage of several cell types through capillary endothelial cells has been documented by *De Bruyn* et al. [1, 7]. Examples of this mechanism include entry of mature blood cells into the peripheral circulation of the bone marrow, entry of lymphocytes into the reticulo-endothelial system, and entry of metastatic myelogenous tumor cells into the circulation. In these instances, the endothelial cells are induced to allow transmural passage, a phenomenon which we have also observed to occur through the flat part of the cells lining Schlemm's canal and the arachnoid villi [19, 20, 22]; in both instances, the channels are temporary.

De Bruyn has shown that, for those regions of the endothelial cells where transmural passage of blood cells, lymphocytes, and tumor cells is possible, the abluminal plasma membrane lacks anionic sialic acid [8]. This suggests a specific mechanism for site recognition. Our preliminary investigations with a cationic cell surface marker (colloidal iron and ferritin, pH 1.3–1.8) showed a dense reaction product along the luminal surface of the endothelial cells lining Schlemm's canal and a weak reaction, irregular binding, and focal absence of sialated glycoproteins along the basal cell surface (fig. 7) [20, 22]. That these regions on the basal cell surface could be pressure-sensitive sites for the formation of unidirectional macrovacuolar configurations, seems likely, and is under further investigation in our laboratory.

The transendothelial channels in the eye and brain, although showing certain similarities to transcellular pathways that occur in other parts of the body and in other species, appear to be unique in the sense that their primary purpose is to provide a dynamic system for bulk outflow of aqueous humor and CSF. Invagination and formation of macrovacuoles differ from those of other endocytotic or 'macropinocytotic' vacuoles in cells where there is internalization of plasma membrane. The formation of vacuoles described here largely implicates an invagination of basal extracellular space, with redistribution or redeployment, rather than massive synthesis, of plasma membrane. At the meeting point of the basal and the apical membranes of the cell, the membranes fuse but this probably

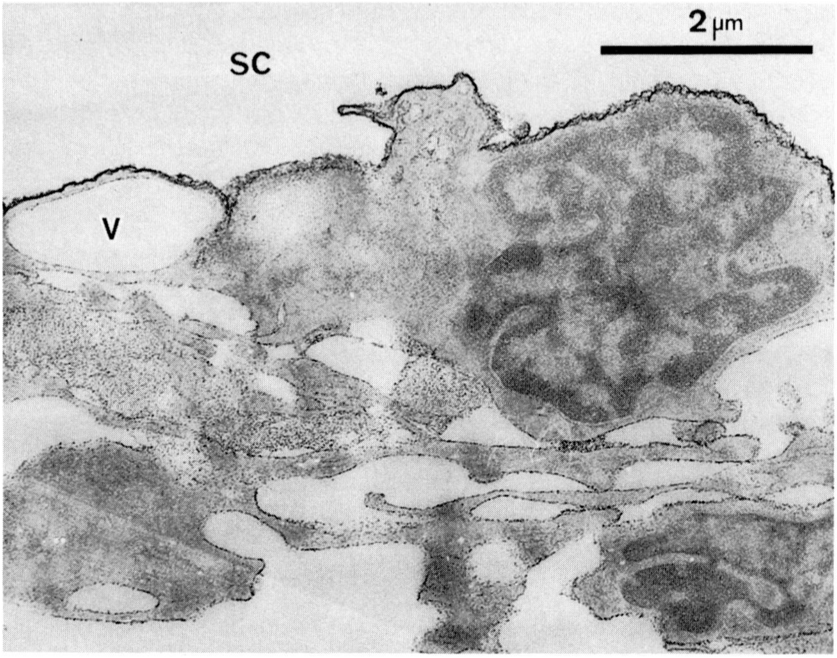

Fig. 7. Electron micrograph of the endothelial lining of Schlemm's canal (SC) and of subendothelial juxtacanalicular tissue. Following glutaraldehyde fixation, the tissue was stained with dialyzed colloidal iron at pH 1.3. Heavy staining is seen on the luminal aspect of the cell, but only a faint and patchy staining reaction is seen on the basal aspect of the cell, as well as along the membrane lining a macrovacuole (V). This indicates the difference in the sialated coating on the two aspects of the cell surface and may contribute to the pressure sensitivity and the consequent formation of unidirectional transcellular channels, i. e., from the basal to the apical direction. Micrograph 14,000 ×.

occurs without loss of plasma membrane. Given the importance of the plasma membrane in the formation of macrovacuolar configurations, it is possible that a disorder of the plasma membrane may lead to a depletion of macrovacuoles, as observed in some cases of chronic simple glaucoma [17, 21, 22]. That such a delicate, pressure-sensitive, one-way valve system should be located in the eye and in the brain is not surprising when one considers the physiologic need for steady-state intraocular and intracranial pressures and metabolic requirements, as well as the need for the bulk outflow of these fluids from their anatomically closed cavities.

Summary

The hydromechanical and metabolic functions of the aqueous humor in the eye and CSF in the brain call for their continuous formation and drainage, the latter taking place by bulk flow. Our investigations in a wide variety of vertebrates have shown that the endothelial lining of the drainage channels, i. e., Schlemm's canal (or analogous structures) in the eye and arachnoid villi/granulations in the brain, is composed of a single layer of flattened cells, with adjacent borders joined by narrow occluding zonules. The bulk outflow of aqueous humor and CSF takes place across the endothelial barrier via a unique dynamic system of vacuolar transcellular channels that are formed through a cyclical sequence of events. The earliest vacuolar configuration originates as a membranous infolding on the basal aspect of the cell surface that gradually enlarges and fuses with the plasma membrane of the apical cell surface; this creates a temporary transendothelial channel through which aqueous humor and CSF escape by mass transfer along a downward pressure gradient, without the need for cellular energy. Morphologic, physiologic, and mechanical evidence indicates that the vacuolar transcellular channels act as a delicate one-way, pressure-sensitive, self-sealing valve system that allows the flow of fluid from the basal to the apical aspect only. We considered various factors, including a pressure-sensitive receptor-mediated mechanism, that may control the formation of these vacuolar transendothelial channels. The endothelial vacuolation cycle, by providing the requisite number of transendothelial pores at any given time, is a chief controlling factor in the maintenance of a steady-state intraocular and intracranial pressure. We have also examined the similarities and dissimilarities of this system to the dynamics of transcellular channels that exist in other vertebrate and invertebrate species.

Acknowledgment

This work was supported in part by a USPHS Award, EY-03747, from the National Eye Institute, Bethesda, Md. Some of the human material was made available through the *Illinois Society for the Prevention of Blindness* and the *National Diabetes Research Interchange.* We appreciate the helpful discussions with Professors *H. Swift, P. De Bruyn, F. Newell,* and *M. LaBarbera* of the University of Chicago and with *S. Vogel* of Duke University.

References

1 Cho, Y.; De Bruyn, P. P. H.: The endothelial structure of the postcapillary venules of the lymph node and the passage of lymphocytes across the venule wall. J. Ultrastruct. Res. *69:* 13–21 (1979).
2 Cole, D. F.: Ocular fluids; in Davson (ed.), The eye, No. 1A, pp. 269–390 (Academic Press, London 1984).
3 Cole, D. F.; Tripathi, R. C.: Theoretical considerations on the mechanism of the aqueous outflow. Expl Eye Res. *12:* 25–30 (1971).
4 Davson, H.: Physiology of the ocular and cerebrospinal fluids (Churchill, London 1956).

5 Davson, H.: Physiology of the cerebrospinal fluid (Churchill, London 1967).
6 Davson, H.: The little brain. Trans. ophthal. Soc. UK *99:* 21–37 (1979).
7 De Bruyn, P. P. H.: Transcellular cell movement and the formation of metastases. Perspect. Biol. Med. *26:* 441–450 (1983).
8 De Bruyn, P. P. H.; Michelson, S.: An anionic material at the advancing front of blood cells entering the bone marrow circulation. Blood *57:* 152–156 (1981).
9 Digby, P. S. B.: Pressure sensitivity and its mechanism in the shallow marine environment. Symp. zool. Soc. Lond. *19:* 159–188 (1967).
10 Evans, E. A.; La Celle, P. L.: Intrinsic material properties of the erythrocyte membrane indicated by mechanical analysis of deformation. Blood *45:* 29–43 (1975).
11 Grierson, I.; Lee, W. R.: Pressure induced changes in the ultrastructure of the endothelium lining Schlemm's canal. Am. J. Ophthal. *80:* 863–884 (1975).
12 Hashimoto, P. H.: Intracellular channels as a route for protein passage in the capillary endothelium of the shark brain. Am. J. Anat. *134:* 41–58 (1972).
13 Knight-Jones, E. W.; Morgan, E.: Responses of marine animals to changes in hydrostatic pressure. Oceanogr. Mar. Biol. Ann. Rev. *4:* 267–299 (1966).
14 Raviola, G.; Raviola, E.: Paracellular route of aqueous outflow in the trabecular meshwork and canal of Schlemm. Investve Ophthal. vis. Sci. *21:* 52–72 (1982).
15 Simionescu, N.; Simionescu, M.; Palade, G. E.: Permeability of muscle capillaries to small heme-peptides. Evidence for the existence of patent transendothelial channels. J. Cell Biol. *64:* 586–607 (1975).
16 Tripathi, R. C.: Mechanism of the aqueous outflow across the trabecular wall of Schlemm's canal. Expl Eye Res. *11:* 116–121 (1971).
17 Tripathi, R. C.: Aqueous outflow pathway in normal and glaucomatous eyes. Br. J. Ophthal. *56:* 157–174 (1972).
18 Tripathi, R. C.: Tracing the bulk outflow route of cerebrospinal fluid by transmission and scanning electron microscopy. Brain Res. *80:* 503–506 (1974).
19 Tripathi, R. C.: Comparative physiology and anatomy of the aqueous outflow pathway; in Davson, Graham (eds.), The eye, No 5, pp. 163–356 (Academic Press, London 1974).
20 Tripathi, R. C.: The functional morphology of the outflow systems of ocular and cerebrospinal fluids; in Bito, Davson, Fenstermacher (eds.), Proc. Fogarty Int. Center Symp., Bethesda 1976. The ocular and cerebrospinal fluids. Expl Eye Res., No 25, suppl., pp. 65–116 (Academic Press, London 1977).
21 Tripathi, R. C.: Pathologic anatomy of the outflow pathway of aqueous humour in chronic simple glaucoma; in Bito, Davson, Fenstermacher (eds.), Proc. Fogarty Int. Center Symp., Bethesda 1976. The ocular and cerebrospinal fluids. Expl Eye Res., No 25, suppl., pp. 403–407 (Academic Press, London 1977).
22 Tripathi, R. C.; Tripathi, B. J.: Functional anatomy of the anterior chamber angle; in Duane (ed.), Biomedical foundations of ophthalmology, No 1, pp. 1–88 (Harper & Row, Philadelphia 1982).
23 Vogel, S.: Evidence for one-way valves in the water-flow system of sponges. J. exp. Biol. *76:* 137– 148 (1978).

R. C. Tripathi, MD, PhD, Eye Research Laboratories, The University of Chicago, 939 East 57th Street, Chicago, IL 60637 (USA)

Prog. appl. Microcirc., vol. 9, pp. 135–136 (Karger, Basel 1985)

Discussion of the Presentation: *Tripathi*

J. Ryan: Is the morphology of your cells any different from that of high endothelium in postcapillary venules, in which the cell appears to be transporting bulk protein? Your cells seem to have many morphological similarities to these high endothelial cells. The reason I state that is, that in certain pathologic conditions, particularly those that have to do with the skin, one finds macrovesicles, very similar to those you described in Schlemm's canal. The cells must obviously have a particular kind of shape in order to cope with this kind of transport, but it can transfer other things besides cells.

R. Tripathi: It's possible and I'm not denying it, because pressure is not the only stimulus that can cause the cell to invaginate and allow the passage. There has to be some kind of receptor, but it looks as though for the endothelial lining of Schlemm's canal that pressure is the determining factor. If we drop the pressure by merely 6–8 mm Hg the vacuoles disappear, yet cells can still migrate through the endothelium although the vacuoles are no longer existent. This suggests that the pressure is probably the primary determining factor, because the eye and the brain have to maintain a steady state of intraocular and intracranial pressure. This is the only pore available to them and so this delicate mechanism is the controlling factor. I agree with you that there could be other mechanisms by which the cell can be indented and a cell can create a passage through another cell.

Casley-Smith: You can see such vacuoles also in injured endothelium, and indeed you can see macromolecules being transferred, but I have never seen such a vacuole open to both sides of the endothelium at once.

R. TRIPATHI: I agree. There is the possibility of macromolecules being transported through the endothelial lining but we find the energy requirement for that will be of such a magnitude that these cells will not be able to provide it. I'm not saying that the vacuolar transcellular channels or the formation of vacuoles may not result due to other stimuli than the pressure. But we are talking here of eye and brain, which represent rather unique structures and we talk about normal situations.

WILLIAMS: The morphology in your scanning electron micrographs of the vacuoles doesn't necessarily suggest a sphere. They are almost reminiscent of what we see in tissue culture when capillaries form tubes. They're somewhat elongated. Could you comment on that?

R. TRIPATHI: That's quite true. These vacuoles are elongated in shape, some of them can be 25 μm in length and they are oriented along the long axis of the cells. Why this configuration occurs to provide an opening at the apical aspect of only about 2.5–3 μm is unknown, but this may be related to the hydrodynamics. These vacuoles are often far from a spheric configuration and some of them take a very sinuous course through the endothelial cell.

END OF DISCUSSION

Prog. appl. Microcirc., vol. 9, pp. 137–143 (Karger, Basel 1985)

Methodology: Especially as it Relates to Theoretical Models of Vesicular Diffusion and Their Implications

St. M. Shea, J. Raskova

Department of Pathology, UMDNJ-Rutgers Medical School, Piscataway, N. J., USA

Introduction

The concept of an endothelial vesicular shuttle as propounded by *Palade* [17] and *Boyles* et al. [2] was first supported by the behavior of tracer substances opaque to electrons as found by *Bruns and Palade* [3]. Later studies with enzymatic tracers by *Karnovsky* [13] and *Simionescu* et al. [23, 24] tended to confirm this interpretation. The shuttle was thought to be specific for macromolecules – for a recent review see *Wagner and Casley-Smith* [26]; it is even suggested by *Williams* [27] that the shuttle may be specific for certain kinds of macromolecules. But the shuttle theory is not without controversy [26], since alternative or complementary structures and functions for plasmalemmal vesicles have been suggested, e. g., by *Bundgaard* et al. [5], by *Simionescu* et al. [24], and by *Clough and Michel* [9]. In our case the appearance of an apparent gradient of labeling of free vesicles – *Karnovsky and Shea* [14], *Johansson* [12] – in response to horseradish peroxidase applied intraluminally or interstitially, encouraged the explicit formulation by *Shea and Karnovsky* [19] of a shuttle model in terms of Brownian motion of the vesicular organelle. This model was later elaborated by *Shea* et al. [20]. The findings of *Casley-Smith and Chin* [6], suggesting that the plasmalemma proves an elastic barrier for vesicles, led to the development of further models allowing for that possibility (*Green and Casley-Smith* [11], *Shea and Bossert* [21]).

Table I. Vesicle diffusion coefficient D_o for a constant cytoplasmic viscosity of one poise

Boltzmann's constant	$k = 1.38 \times 10^{-16}$ deg mole
Absolute temperature	$T = 310$ °K
Cytoplasmic viscosity	$\eta = 1$ Poise
Vesicle radius	$a = 30$ nm
Diffusion coefficient	$D_o = \frac{kT}{6\pi a \eta}$
	$= 7.565 \times 10^{-10}$ cm^2 s^{-1} for $\eta = 1$ P

Table II. Vesicular transport by Brownian motion with a constant cytoplasmic diffusion coefficient and absorbing barriers: theoretical values

Cell width	300 nm
Vesicle radius	30 nm
Diffusion distance, W	240 nm
Starting position, Y	20 nm
Transit time	126.01 ms/P
Retreating time	20.22 ms/P
Sojourn time	29.04 ms/P
Fractional transiting vesicle flux, ϕ_R	$0.08\dot{3}$

Table III. Vesicular transport by Brownian motion with the effective diffusion coefficient modified by hydraulic forces and absorption determined by cut-off points close to the walls by *London-van der Waals* forces[1]

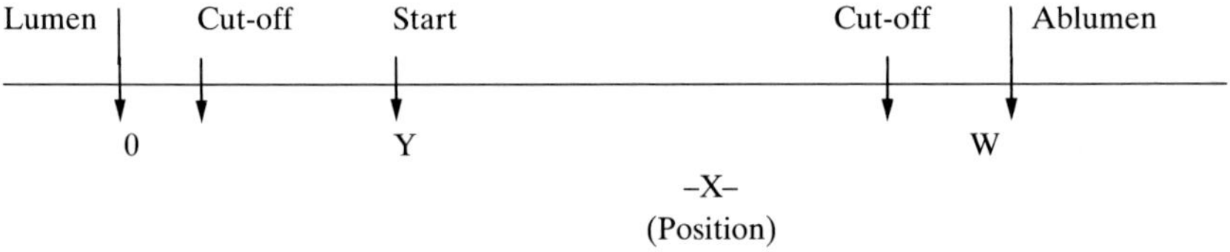

Cell width	300 nm
Vesicle radius, R	30 nm
Diffusion distance, W	240 nm
Starting position, Y	20 nm
Van der Waals cut-off points	1.5 nm from walls

[1] *Weinbaum and Caro* [28]

However, it is the development of new models by *Weinbaum and Caro* [28] and by *Arminski* et al. [1], in which the effective diffusion coefficient is no longer regarded as constant but as being modified by hydraulic interaction with the plasmalemma, which seems most relevant to current methodology. To make the findings of *Weinbaum and Caro* [28] more readily accessible to experimentalists, we have devised a method of exploring their results for arbitrary parameters by Monte Carlo computer simulation.

Methods

This model [28] retains a constant distance of release of the free vesicle from the plasmalemma, as in *Shea* et al. [20] (see diagram in table III), and replaces the plasmalemma as an absorbing barrier by cut-off points close to the plasmalemma determined by short-ranged London-van der Waals attractive forces (*Weinbaum and Caro* [28]). The approximate variation in the cytosol diffusion coefficient ascribed to hydraulic forces by *Weinbaum and Caro* [28] is shown in table IV, along with its implementation in the simulation. This approximation [28] has been shown to be quite good by a more exact treatment by *Arminski* et al. [1]. Simulations of vesicular diffusion with a constant diffusion coefficient, by *Shea* et al. [20] and by *Shea and Raskova* [22], have proved accurate, in relation to exact computed values as listed in table II.

For example, in a recent test used as a 'benchmark' for our pseudorandom number generator, where the fractional transiting flux is theoretically $\phi_R = 0.0833$, simulation gave a result of $\phi_R = 0.0842$.

The actual simulations were carried out as indicated in tables IV and V. The only difficulty encountered was the necessity to use a very short time increment to obtain convergence on a stable solution. This is, apparently, the random walk equivalent of a counterintuitive finding of *Feller* [10] in the case of the 'gambler's ruin problem', that, 'if the stakes are doubled while the initial capital remains unchanged, the probability of ruin decreases for the player whose probability of success is $P < 1/2$ and increases for the adversary (for whom the game is advantageous)'.

Results

Results are tabulated in tables I–VI. Note the increase in times listed in table VI over those in table II. The fractional transiting flux, ϕ_R, was 0.156 ± 0.023, SE computed from *Snedecor and Cochrane* [25]. This is not significantly different from the value of approximately 0.180 shown in figure 8 by *Weinbaum and Caro* [28] for a geometrically very similar model with identical cut-off distances.

Table IV. Approximate correction of diffusion coefficient to allow for hydrodynamic interaction of the vesicle with the plasmalemma in the computation of vesicle displacement[1]

$$\lambda = 1 + {}^{R}/_{X} + {}^{R}/_{(W-X)}$$

$$D = D_o/_\lambda$$

The value of a pseudorandom number uniformly distributed between 0 and 1 determines whether the displacement is positive or negative. The mean of two consecutive (Δ_1X, Δ_2X) such displacements is taken in computing the effect of λ and D.

[1] *Weinbaum and Caro* [28]

Table V. Simulation of vesicle displacement

Δt	$= 0.0033$ ms				
For D	$= D_o$	Δ_1X	$= \pm \sqrt{2D_o\Delta t}$ per poise	$= \pm$	0.70711 nm
For D	$= D_o/_\lambda$	Δ_1X		$= \pm$	$0.70711/\sqrt{\lambda_1}$ nm
		Δ_2X		$= \pm$	$0.70711/\sqrt{\lambda_2}$ nm
		ΔX		$=$	$(\Delta_1X + \Delta_2X)/2$

where X = vesicle position at time t, $X_n = X_{n-1} \pm \Delta X$, $t_n = t_{n-1} + \Delta t$, where $\pm\, \Delta X$ is calculated according to table IV from $\pm\, (\Delta_1X + \Delta_2X)/2$

Table VI. Simulation of vesicular transport with variable cytoplasmic viscosity in a cell 300 nm thick

(a)	Number of vesicles traversing cell	39
(b)	Number of vesicles retreating	211
(c)	Average traversal time of (a)	$2683 \times \eta$ ms
(d)	Average retreating time of (b)	$112 \times \eta$ ms
(e)	Average sojourn of vesicles (a) and (b)	$513 \times \eta$ ms

Discussion

Comparison of the free vesicle sojourn times of tables II and VI gives an estimate of the relative free vesicle concentrations required to sustain vesicular transport. Assuming symmetrical vesicular shuttling from both sides, from the results of *Shea and Bossert* [21] a transiting flux of

1 vesicle/($\mu m^2 \cdot s$) would be maintained by a free vesicle concentration, over the diffusion region, of 2.954 vesicles/($\mu m^3 \eta$). Since the sojourn times of tables VI and II are in the ratio of 17.67, this suggests a corresponding increase in the free vesicle concentration required to sustain a transiting flux of 1 vesicle/($\mu m^2 \cdot s$). However, since the values of ϕ_R from tables II and VI are respectively 0.0833 and 0.156, the actual ratio is 9.44, i.e., the increase in free vesicle concentration required is only to 27.88 vesicles/($\mu m^3 \eta$). For the vesicular transiting flux suggested by *Renkin* [18] of 3 vesicles/($\mu m^2 \cdot s$) this would amount to a concentration of 83.63 free vesicles/($\mu m^3 \eta$); this also assumes a capillary surface density of $7 \times 10^3 cm^2/100\,g$ [18]. If the higher capillary endothelial surface density of $2 \times 10^4 cm^2/100\,g$ of *Casley-Smith* et al. [7] is assumed, a free vesicle concentration of 29 vesicles/($\mu m^3 \eta$) would be required.

Clearly, much depends on the accurate estimation of at least two of the three variables: cytoplasmic viscosity, concentration of free vesicles, and vesicular transit time. Of these three, the estimates of cytoplasmic viscosity are the most questionable. The estimate of 8.9 P by *Arminski* et al. [1] is based on transient labeling experiments on thick cardiac endothelial and on mesothelial cells by *Casley-Smith and Chin* [6], and on the questionable velocity of fixation by glutaraldehyde as shown by *Buckley* [4]. Another estimate of 8 P by *Shea* et al. [20] is even more indirect. However, an upper limit on the vesicular transit time for rat cardiac capillary endothelium, using horseradish peroxidase, of about 6–9 s has been obtained by *Boyles* et al. [2]; this would, accordingly, suggest an upper limit on viscosity of the order of 2.2 – 3.35 P, on the basis of the transit time of 2.68(ηs) of table VI. Given the assumptions considered above as to vesicular transit flux and capillary endothelial surface density [7, 18], this would entail a free vesicle concentration of about 64–98 free vesicles/ μm^3.

Low estimates of the concentration of free vesicles are based on glutaraldehyde fixation, which is notoriously slow – see [2, 4]. Contrary conclusions can be based on experiments using a ruthenium red tracer and a fixative containing acrolein, done by *Chien* et al. [8], who estimate that 8.15% of aortic endothelial vesicles are free. In rapidly frozen rabbit lung *Mazzone* et al. [15] estimated that in lung capillaries about 100 vesicles/ (μm^3) are free (see their fig. 6). A similar conclusion is suggested by the finding of *McGuire and Twietmeyer* [16] that rapid freezing of aortic endothelial cells reduces the number of caveolae to about 30% of those observed in glutaraldehyde-fixed material with or without freezing.

Summary

The study of theoretical models suggests that the best targets for methodological attention are experimental estimates of the free vesicle concentration and of the vesicle transit time. Freezing methods would appear preferable to chemical methods of fixation in both cases. It would be ideal if the enzymatic methods of *Boyles* et al. [2] could feasibly be combined with freezing methods to arrest vesicular motion and obtain an accurate estimate of the transit time, if indeed a shuttle process occurs. Similarly, a synthesis of the theory of a shuttle process with the theory of transient vesicular fusions with exchange of contents put forward by *Clough and Michel* [9] seems conceivable, given the time-scale contemplated; the only difficulty here is the considerable early labeling of abluminal vesicles they report [9], though this may be peculiar to the frog. Any estimates of cytoplasmic viscosity are clearly dependent on more directly accessible observables.

References

1 Arminski, L.; Weinbaum, S.; Pfeffer, R.: Time dependent theory of vesicular transport across endothelium. J. theor. Biol. *85:* 13–43 (1980).
2 Boyles, J.; L'Hernault, N.; Laks, H.; Palade, G. E.: Evidence for vesicular shuttle in heart capillaries. J. Cell Biol. *91:* 418a (1981).
3 Bruns, R. R.; Palade, G. E.: Studies on blood capillaries. II. Transport of ferritin molecules across the wall of muscle capillaries. J. Cell Biol. *37:* 277–299 (1968).
4 Buckley, I. K.: Studies in fixation for electron microscopy using cultured cells. Lab. Invest. *29:* 398–410 (1973).
5 Bundgaard, M.; Frøkjær-Jensen, J.; Crone, C.: Endothelial plasmalemmal vesicles as elements in a system of branching invaginations from the cell surface. Proc. natn. Acad. Sci. USA *76:* 6439–6449 (1979).
6 Casley-Smith, J. R.; Chin, J. C.: The passage of endothelial vesicles across endothelial and mesothelial cells. J. Microscopy, Oxford *93:* 167–189 (1971).
7 Casley-Smith, J. R.; Green, H. S.; Harris, J. L.; Wadey, P. J.: The quantitative morphology of skeletal muscles in relation to permeability. Microvasc. Res. *10:* 43–64 (1975).
8 Chien, S.; Laufer, L.; Handley, D. A.: Vesicle distribution in the arterial endothelium determined with ruthenium red as an extracellular marker. J. Ultrastruct. Res. *79:* 198–206 (1982).
9 Clough, G.; Michel, C. C.: The role of vesicles in the transport of ferritin through frog endothelium. J. Physiol., Lond. *315:* 127–142 (1981).
10 Feller, W.: An introduction to probability theory and its implications; vol. I, 2nd ed., pp. 311–317 (Wiley, New York, London 1950).
11 Green, H. S.; Casley-Smith, J. R.: Calculation on the passage of small vesicles across endothelial cells by Brownian motion. J. theor. Biol. *35:* 103–111 (1972).
12 Johansson, B. R.: Permeability of muscles capillaries to interstitially injected horseradish peroxidase. Microvasc. Res. *16:* 340–353 (1978).
13 Karnovsky, M. J.: Vesicular transport of exogenous peroxidase across capillary endothelium into the T-system of muscle. J. Cell Biol. *27:* 49A–50A (1965).

14 Karnovsky, M. J.; Shea, S. M.: Transcapillary transport by pinocytosis. Microvasc. Res. *2:* 353–360 (1970).
15 Mazzone, R. W.; Kornblau, S. M.: Pinocytotic vesicles in endothelium of rapidly frozen rabbit lung. Microvasc. Res. *21:* 193–211 (1981).
16 McGuire, P. G.; Twietmeyer, T. A.: Morphology of rapidly frozen aortic endothelial cells. Glutaraldehyde fixation increases the number of caveolae. Circulation Res. *53:* 424–429 (1983).
17 Palade, G. E.: Transport in quanta across the endothelium of blood capillaries. Anat. Rec. *136:* 254 (1960).
18 Renkin, E. M.: Multiple pathways of capillary permeability. Circulation Res. *41:* 735–743 (1977).
19 Shea, S. M.; Karnovsky, M. J.: Brownian motion: a theoretical explanation for the movement of vesicles across the endothelium. Nature, Lond. *212:* 353–356 (1966).
20 Shea, S. M.; Karnovsky, M. J.; Bossert, W. H.: Vesicular transport across endothelium: Simulation of a diffusion model. J. theor. Biol. *24:* 30–42 (1969).
21 Shea, S. M.; Bossert, W. H.: Vesicular transport across endothelium: A generalized diffusion model. Microvasc. Res. *6:* 305–315 (1973).
22 Shea, S. M.; Raskova, J.: Vesicular diffusion and thermal forces. Fed. Proc. *42:* 2431–2434 (1982).
23 Simionescu, N.; Simionescu, M.; Palade, G. E.: Permeability of muscle capillaries to exogenous myoglobin. J. Cell Biol. *57:* 424–452 (1973).
24 Simionescu, N.; Simionescu, M.; Palade, G. E.: Permeability of muscle capillaries to small heme-peptides. J. Cell Biol. *64:* 586–607 (1975).
25 Snedecor, G. W.; Cochrane, W. G.: Statistical methods. 6th ed.; pp. 327–329. (Iowa State, Ames, Iowa, 1972).
26 Wagner, R. C.; Casley-Smith, J. R.: Review: Endothelial vesicles. Microvasc. Res. *21:* 267–298 (1981).
27 Williams, S. K.: Vesicular transport of proteins by capillary endothelium. Ann. N. Y. Acad. Sci. *416:* 457–467 (1984).
28 Weinbaum, S.; Caro, C. G.: A macromolecular transport model for the arterial wall and endothelium based on the ultrastructural specialization observed in electron microscopical studies. J. fluid Mech. *74:* 611–640 (1976).

Stephen M. Shea, MD, Department of Pathology, UMDNJ-Rutgers Medical School, Piscataway, NJ 08854 (USA)

Prog. appl. Microcirc., vol. 9, pp. 144–145 (Karger, Basel 1985)

Discussion of the Presentation: *Shea*

CASLEY-SMITH: Instead of *Weinbaum and Caro*'s model, it's much easier to employ the model that *Green* and I used, where you simply have an alpha for probability of a vesicle not fusing and then you can ascribe it to the *van der Waal*'s forces.

SHEA: I think you and I did the same thing. We invented a phenomenological reflection coefficient to account for the embarassing numbers but now the numbers are in question.

TAYLOR: I don't want to leave you with the impression that I think the vesicles transport anything across membranes. I was trying to think of ways that they might do it, but what they must do is to produce four populations like we've shown in many organs. In addition, there is no doubt that most of this is volume-mediated flow as Dr. CRONE was pointing out, which I didn't understand at the time, or you wouldn't get these reflection coefficients around 0.9. I know you are trying to do it with time, but you have to have selectivity as well as turnover time in order to explain the tremendous amount of data that we now have.

SHEA: I think that topic should be addressed by Drs. WAGNER or WILLIAMS. I'm not saying that all macromolecules will be treated as equal by the vesicles. But if you have data on a given macromolecule, then you could make some computations as to whether the vesicles could actually account for the flow. I thought that you were leaving open the possibility that reflection coefficients of less than one could admit of some of the macromolecules or a lot of them going across as Dr. RENKIN suggested this morning by a ferry boat mechanism of some sort.

TAYLOR: I really thought I kept the probability of transendothelial vesicular transport but I was very cautious, because many people don't think there are such things. But that's very tempting, because it gives you both large and small pore possibilities. By small I mean 45 Å. It also fits the data with positive charge that we see with lymph to plasma measurements.

FRØKJÆR-JENSEN: Could you please tell me the difference in mathematical treatment between formation of channels between two separate systems and a few vesicles moving a very short distance from one system to another, instead of from one front to the other front?

SHEA: I think the difference would be simply that the diffusion distance would be shortened and that the calculations would have to be adjusted. But since you would be dealing with a statistical average of some kind I think the computations would be horrendous. In addition, I think that Dr. MICHEL's model would pose similar difficulties for the mathematician.

MICHEL: Could I raise a quick point, and that is that there is some experimental evidence against vesicles acting as shuttles, moving from one surface to another surface. If you label the plasmalemmal membrane it's not transmitted with the vesicles, whereas the tracers appear to move from vesicle to vesicle. Dr. CLOUGH also showed with cationized ferritin that the luminal caveolae themselves, i.e., their membrane doesn't appear to be transmitted.

SHEA: That would fit with the ideas of the *Simionescus*. There is, however, another problem: In the iris there is some evidence of an unidirectional transport of material. If this is true, then the question becomes very serious 'how would the membrane ever get back'? You would have to invent a membrane flow theory. But if the *Simionescus* are right, this membrane flow theory wouldn't be available to you. Somebody's got to be wrong somewhere.

END OF DISCUSSION

Prog. appl. Microcirc., vol. 9, pp. 146–149 (Karger, Basel 1985)

Characterization of Anionic Microdomains on Luminal Vesicles in Rat Pulmonary Capillary Endothelium

S. Villaschi[a], *L. Johns, G. G. Pietra*

Department of Pathology and Laboratory Medicine, University of Pennsylvania Medical School, Philadelphia, Pa., USA

[a] Dr. Villaschi is recipient of a NATO fellowship from the University of Rome, Italy

Introduction

Endothelial cells play an active role in molecular traffic between blood and interstitium. This requires the ability of the endothelium to discriminate molecules not only on the basis of size but also of structure. Selectivity may be due in part to the presence of anionic microdomains contributed by glycoproteins and glycosaminoglycans strategically located on the endothelial surface [7]. In studying the topography of these domains in the lung microvascular endothelium, we have recently observed the existence of two populations of luminal endothelial vesicles. One group of vesicles was apparently devoid of anionic sites, the other contained highly charged anionic regions [5]. In the present study, we have found that these anionic sites on luminal endothelial vesicles are rich in heparan sulfate. We suggest that they may represent specialized regions of the endothelium for interaction with circulating substances [5, 6].

Material and Methods

Experiments were performed on anesthetized and artificially ventilated female, Sprague-Dawley rats wt. 200–250 g. High charge density anionic sites were identified ultrastructurally using cationized ferritin (CF) (P. I. 9.3–9.5) in perfusate containing high salt molarities (0.2–0.5 M $MgCl_2$) as described previously [5]. The experimental protocol is summarized in table I.

Table I. Protocol for localization of high charge density anionic sites in the lung microvascular endothelium*

Treatment	Dose	Time (min)	Temp. °C	pH
$MgCl_2$	0.2–0.5 M	1.5–5	37	7.4
NaCl	0.15M	5	4	7.4
NaCl	0.15M	5	37	7.4
Fixation**	2%	40	37	7.2
Pronase	2.5 U/ml	10	30	7.4
Neuraminidase	2.0 U/ml	60	37	5.5
Heparinase	20 U/ml	60	38	7.0
Heparitinase	50 U/ml	60	38	7.0
Chondroitinase ABC	1.5 U/ml	60	37	7.4
Chondroitinase AC	1.5 U/ml	60	37	7.4

* Enzymes were perfused in appropriate buffers containing 4% BSA except for pronase where BSA was replaced by 4% Dextran 80. Pronase and chondroitinase were perfused in Hank's balanced salt solution. Heparinase, heparitinase and neuraminidase were perfused in acetate buffer. Controls were perfused in buffers without enzymes.
** 1% paraformaldehyde–1% glutaraldehyde in 0.1 M cacodylate buffer. Free aldehydes were quenched with 0.5 M NH_4Cl.

Table II. Removal of high charge density anionic sites after perfusion of rat lung with purified heparinase and purified heparitinase*

Treatment	% Decorated Vesicles (Mean ± SD)	Reduction (%)	p
Control (0.2 M $MgCl_2$)	58.00 ± 10.00	–	–
Heparinase	30.95 ± 5.74	46.64	< 0.001
Heparitinase	35.86 ± 5.50	38.17	< 0.005

* The data are based on three animals per treatment. For each experimental condition, measurements were made on 25 capillaries in sections cut from 4–6 blocks chosen at random from the midthird of the left lung.

Results

In the presence of high salt molarities (0.2–0.5 M $MgCl_2$) CF was bound only to the stomata and stomatal diaphragms of 58 ± 10 SD % luminal vesicles (table II). Decoration of the vesicles was not altered by prefixation of lungs with aldehydes but it was completely abolished by preperfusion with pronase. Purified heparinase or purified heparitinase significantly ($p < 0.005$) decreased the population of labeled vesicles (table II) as compared to controls. Neuraminidase, chondroitinase ABC and chondroitinase AC had no apparent effect.

Discussion

This study indicates that endothelial vesicles in the rat pulmonary capillaries can be subdivided into two classes on the basis of their ability to bind electrostatically CF. It is likely that this phenomenon is not unique to the rat lung but may be shared by other microvascular endothelia. The physiologic significance of this organization is unknown but the presence of heparan sulfate suggests a role for interaction with circulating macromolecules. Among these, lipoproteins and chylomicrons are major candidates since heparan sulfate links lipoprotein lipase to the endothelial cell [3], and very low density lipoproteins [4] and chylomicra [2] are catabolized by the lung endothelium. Other possibilities include interaction with clotting factors [1].

We speculate that the two populations of endothelial vesicles may reflect functional differentiation of the pulmonary endothelium. Vesicles rich in heparan sulfate could be the sites of interactions with circulating substrates. Vesicles devoid of exposed anionic sites may represent transcapillary routes for anionic macromolecules.

Summary

Luminal vesicles in the pulmonary microvascular endothelium are heterogeneous in their complement of anionic sites. About half of the vesicles contain high charge density anionic sites rich in heparan sulfate, the other half has no detectable anionic sites. The two populations may serve different functions, heparan sulfate-rich vesicles may be the sites for interaction with circulating substrates, vesicles devoid of exposed anionic sites may serve instead to transport anionic plasma proteins.

Acknowledgment

This research was supported in part by Grant HL-32482 from the NHBLI.

References

1 Buonassisi, V.; Colburn, P.: Antibodies to the heparan sulfate proteoglycans synthesized by endothelial cell cultures. Biochim. biophys. Acta *760* : 1–12 (1983).

2 Hamosh, M.; Yeager, H. Jr.; Shechter, Y.; Hamosh, P.: Lipoprotein lipase in rat lung. Effect of dexamethasone. Biochim. biophys. Acta *431* : 519–525 (1976).

3 Olivecrona, T.; Bengtsson, G.; Marklung, S. E.; Lindahl, U.; Höök, N.: Heparin-lipoprotein lipase interactions. Fed Proc. *36* : 60–65 (1977).

4 Pietra, G. G.; Spagnoli, L. G.; Capuzzi, D. M.; Sparks, C. E.; Fishman, A. P.; Marsh, J. B.: Metabolism of ^{125}I–labeled lipoproteins by the isolated rat lung. J. Cell Biol. *70* : 33–46 (1976).

5 Pietra, G. G.; Sampson, P.; Lanken, P. N.; Hansen-Flaschen, J.; Fishman, A. P.: Transcapillary movement of cationized ferritin in the isolated perfused rat lung. Lab. Invest. *49* : 54–61 (1983).

6 Ryan, U. S.: Structural bases for metabolic activity. Annu. Rev. Physiol. *44:* 223–239 (1982).

7 Simionescu, N.; Simionescu, M.; Palade, G. E.: Differentiated microdomains on the luminal surface of the capillary endothelium. I. Preferential distribution of anionic sites. J. Cell Biol. *90* : 605–613 (1981).

G. G. Pietra, MD, Anatomic Pathology Division, Hospital of the University of Pennsylvania, 34th and Spruce Streets, Philadelphia, PA 19104 (USA)

Prog. appl. Microcirc., vol. 9, pp. 150–164 (Karger, Basel 1985)

Use of Endothelial Cells in Culture for Studies of the Microcirculation

U. S. Ryan

Department of Medicine D-58, University of Miami, School of Medicine, Miami, Fla., USA

Introduction

Most studies of the microcirculation, of microvascular endothelial cells, and of microvascular endothelial cell vesicles, are directed towards understanding mechanisms for transport of water and macromolecules across the endothelial barrier. As a result most studies of endothelial vesicles have focused on their possible role in these processes.

Our studies, on the other hand, have a completely different vantage point. Our long term goal has been to try to understand the processing of vasoactive substances during circulation through the lungs. These studies have led to examination of the smallest vessels where reactions between blood-borne substrates and endothelial cells would be expected to occur most efficiently. At the level of the pulmonary capillaries the endothelial cells are endowed, as are endothelial cells elsewhere, with vesicles, or caveolae; many of which directly face the vascular lumen. Previous studies using isolated perfused blood-free rat lungs indicate that substances such as the adenine nucleotides, and oligopeptide hormones such as bradykinin and angiotensin I, are metabolized quantitatively during one passage through the lungs. Studies using techniques of cytochemistry at the electron microscope level indicate that the enzymes responsible for the processing of the adenine nucleotides are localized within endothelial caveolae. Immunocytochemical studies demonstrate that angiotensin converting enzyme, the enzyme responsible both for metabolism of bradykinin and for conversion of angiotensin I to angiotensin II, is localized on both undifferentiated portions of the plasma membrane and on the caveola membranes. Thus, caveolae clearly have the effect of increasing the luminal surface area of the endothelium and, therefore, of the enzymes available for processing, but may also provide a specialized microenvironment in direct communication with the vascular space.

We have now examined a number of endothelial surface enzymes using cell cultures, a condition where transport across the endothelial layer is of no physiological significance and is unlikely to occur. Endothelial cultures have the advantage that enzymatic contributions from other cell types or from the blood can be ruled out and the additional advantage that substances can be introduced into the medium above the cells and the metabolites released back into the medium can be analyzed with ease. Endothelial cell cultures allow examination of shape changes, and responses of endothelial cells to injurious or specific stimuli without conferring additional or related changes to an intact vessel or animal preparation. Under such conditions, we have found that the vesicular system may be internalized in response to changes in cell shape and to noxious stimuli in such a way that it may also function to protect and 'bank' endothelial enzymes, so that they can be returned to the surface rapidly and without requiring new synthesis or re-insertion into the cell membranes.

Endothelial Cell Culture

Methods for isolation, identification, and culture of endothelial cells from the lungs are now routine [16, 17]. A number of different methods are available for obtaining large vessel endothelium, and endothelium from the microvasculature, using digestion with enzymes such as collagenase [19, 29]. While these methods are widely used and have served a useful purpose in establishing a field of endothelial cell culture and in defining a number of endothelial properties [15, 29], they are not without hazard. Proteolytic enzymes, particularly trypsin and tryptic contaminants of collagenase, damage endothelial cells during the harvesting procedure by removing receptors, enzymes, and junctional proteins from the surface [8, 22, 23]. The most serious effects of exposure of cells to trypsin are likely to be encountered when endothelial cells are passaged by standard procedures using trypsin/EDTA mixtures [19]. Thus, repeated treatment with trypsin may be a factor in the in vitro 'aging' of endothelial cell cultures [22] and may produce changes in the surface properties of endothelial cells that render them more adherent for each other [2] and for circulating immune complexes [23].

New techniques that avoid exposure to proteolytic enzymes during either isolation or during subculture have now been developed [16]. Cells are removed by mechanical scraping and can be scaled up for long-term, large-scale culture using microcarriers [21]. The microcarriers can also be used as a means for collecting pulmonary microvascular endothelial cells, either from the pre-capillary vessels [30] on the arterial side or from the post-capillary vessels on the venous side [28]. Cultures that have never been exposed to proteolytic enzymes can be maintained in large quantities for long periods (several years) without losing phenotypic characteristics. They have the advantage that multiple experiments can be performed on one cell line, obviating the necessity for determining base-line measurements on each new isolate.

Once an endothelial cell line is established in culture it can be used for a number of functional and structural studies with far greater ease than could be performed on endothelial cells in situ in an intact animal, organ or single vessel preparation. Furthermore, influences that cannot be attributed to endothelium per se can be ruled out. However, it is worth mentioning that culture is itself an artificial situation and the cells are deprived of their normal relationships with circulating blood cells and plasma components and with other cell types of the vascular wall. It is necessary to validate all data obtained, using endothelial cells in culture, with data obtained in vivo. It is also necessary to monitor cultures for the continuing presence of properties characteristic of the cell-type in vivo [26].

Functional Properties of Endothelial Caveolae

The adenine nucleotides are inactivated during passage through the lungs [3, 7, 12]. The metabolism is not dependent on blood enzymes and does not involve uptake into cells of the lungs or pulmonary vessels, but clearly occurs at a site where the substrates circulating in the blood are able to interact with cellular enzymes and immediately return the metabolic products to the blood stream [12, 33]. Electron microscope cytochemistry (carried out on intact perfused lungs) shows this site to be the luminal caveolae of endothelial cells of the pulmonary microcirculation [32, 33]. However, when blocks of fixed lung are used, all caveolae (luminal and abluminal) appear to contain enzymes [33]. Clearly, therefore, endothelial caveolae are not only ideally positioned to process circulating adenine nucleotides and to return the degradation products to the circulation, but also possess the requisite enzymes. In vivo, only those enzymes that have access to substrate take part in processing, but caveolae on the abluminal surface of the endothelial cell also contain enzymes.

The cytochemical localization of 5′-nucleotidase within endothelial caveolae allowed development of a rapid, simple means of obtaining an endothelial plasma membrane-caveolae fraction from the lungs [11, 12, 34]. This fraction is capable of inactivating the adenine nucleotides to adenosine and free phosphate [11, 12], of inactivating bradykinin and converting angiotensin I to angiotensin II ([14] and see below).

We, therefore, began to examine for the cellular and subcellular sites of the enzymes responsible for the metabolism of the kinins and angiotensins.

In earlier studies we had shown that bradykinin is inactivated and that angiotensin I is converted to angiotensin II in a single pass through the pulmonary circulation [18]. The same enzyme, angiotensin converting enzyme (ACE), also known as kininase II, is responsible for both reactions. Using intrinsically labeled components it could be argued from the kinetics of disappearance, that bradykinin and angiotensin were metabolized on or close to the luminal surface of blood vessels. Using isolated endothelial cells on cellulose acetate paper, it became clear that endothelial cells alone were responsible for the pulmonary metabolism of these compounds [13], and using plasma membrane fractions the endothelial caveolae were directly implicated [14]. Since the kinetics of disappearance of the adenine nucleotides and the polypeptide hormones, bradykinin and angiotensin I, are similar, it is not surprising that the sites of their degradative enzymes are also similar. Using antibodies to angiotensin converting enzyme, immunocytochemistry at the EM level indicates that the enzyme is localized on the plasma membrane, including caveolae, of pulmonary endothelial cells of the lungs (fig. 1 c).

The ability of endothelial cells isolated as Häutchen preparations on cellulose acetate paper to conduct reactions yielding products similar to those obtained using intact perfused lungs, indicates that the metabolism of bradykinin and conversion of angiotensin I to angiotensin II is a property of endothelial cells. With the advent of techniques for culture of pulmonary endothelial cells it became possible to show not only that endothelial cells freshly removed from vessels possess this property, but that the cells are capable of synthesizing the enzyme [19], and of inserting it in the plasma membrane such that its active site is accessible to circulating substrates. Immunocytochemical localizations, using endothelial cells

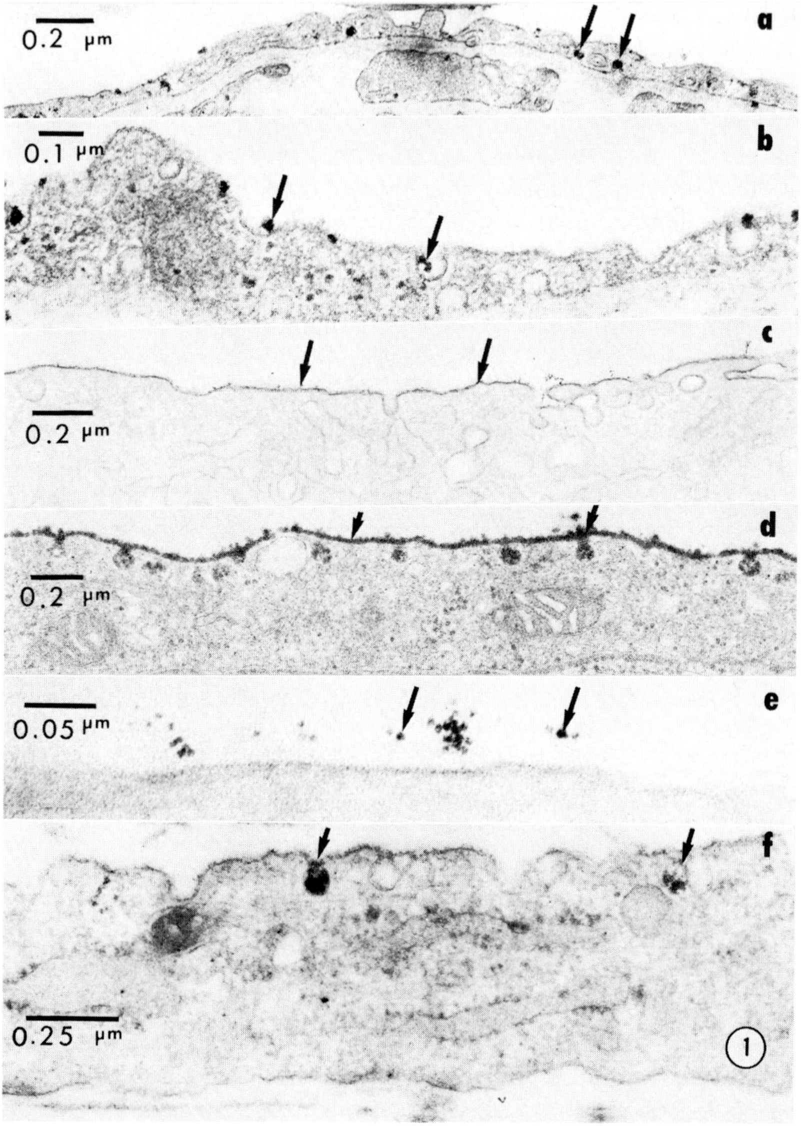

Fig. 1. This figure illustrates some of the enzymes of the endothelial plasma membrane and associated caveolae. *a* shows the cytochemical localization of ATPase on a capillary endothelial cell of fixed rat lung incubated with lead nitrate and ATP. Reaction product, indicating sites of ATPase activity, is specifically localized in caveolae (arrows). *b* shows the

that have been maintained in culture for many months, indicate that the subcellular site of the enzyme is on the plasma membrane and on those caveolae that are confluent with the exterior (fig. 1 c).

On account of the ease with which cells in culture can be used to investigate endothelial properties, there is now a long list of enzymes, enzyme inhibitors, receptors, transport proteins and hemostatic factors associated with endothelial cells. Some of these properties have been shown to be due to products synthesized by endothelial cells, others seem to be properties of the endothelial surface acquired by contact with plasma.

A priori, rapid reactions occurring at the endothelial surface are likely to be due to structures situated on the cell surface. However, the cellular response to binding of specific molecules at the surface of the cell frequently elicits an intracellular response, e.g., the bradykinin stimulated release of PGI_2, [4, 5] and rise in adenylate and guanylate cyclase [20].

Advances in endothelial cell culture techniques have been paralleled by technical improvements in assays suitable for use with small numbers of cells [10]. Sometimes the assay technology can be used for making comparable in vivo measurements [9]. In addition, there is a growing list of antibodies available against endothelial substances. Carbonic anhydrase, an enzyme responsible for facilitating removal of CO_2 from plasma bicarbonate and in maintaining blood pH; alpha 2 macroglobulin, an enzyme

---

cytochemical localization of 5′-nucleotidase on a capillary endothelial cell of rat lung perfused blood-free in situ, then perfused with lead nitrate and AMP. Sites of 5′-nucleotidase activity are localized on caveolae facing the vascular lumen (arrows). *c* shows the immunocytochemical localization of ACE on a pulmonary endothelial cell in culture. Cells were incubated unfixed with antibodies to ACE then with a secondary antibody conjugated to peroxidase. The peroxidase moiety was reacted with 3,3′-diaminobenzidine in the presence of H_2O_2. The electron-dense reaction product indicating sites of immunoreactive ACE (arrows) is localized along the plasma membrane, including caveolae. *d* shows the immunocytochemical localization of CPN. Bovine pulmonary artery endothelial cells were incubated with antibodies to bovine plasma carboxypeptidase N and then treated as in *c*. Reaction product is on the plasma membrane and associated caveolae (arrows). *e* shows the immunocytochemical localization of carbonic anhydrase. Bovine pulmonary endothelial cells were incubated with antibodies to carbonic anhydrase, then with secondary antibodies conjugated to ferritin. Sites of reactivity (arrows) are localized on the plasma membrane, the ferritin tag is restricted by a layer approximately 100 Å thick. *f* shows immunocytochemical localization of calmodulin, reaction product is indicated by an arrow, not all caveolae are labeled. Bar markers (*a*) 0.2 μm, (*b*) 0.1 μm, (*c*) 0.2 μm, (*d*) 0.2 μm, (*e*) 0.05 μm, (*f*) 0.25 μm.

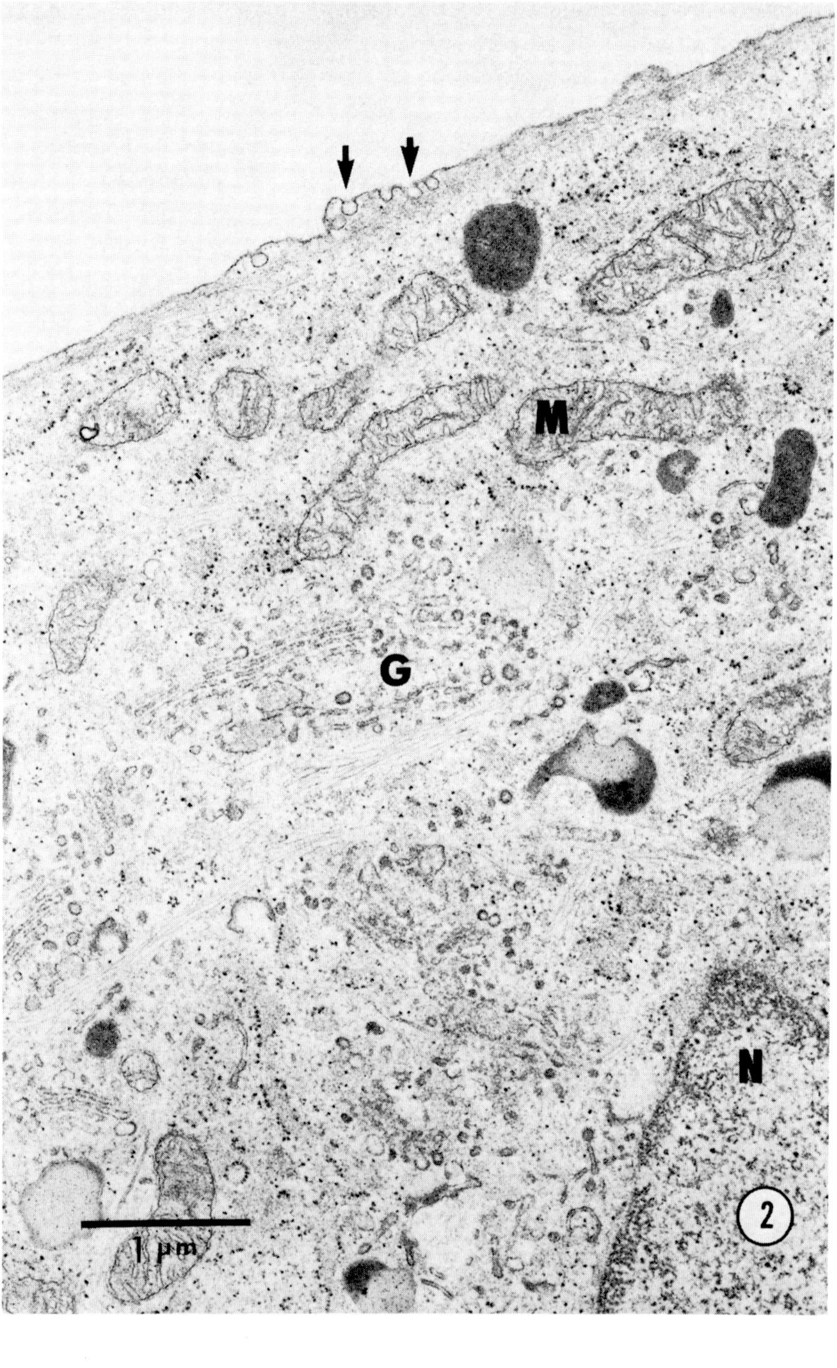
M
G
N
1 µm
2

inhibitor; carboxypeptidase N (CPN), an enzyme that may be important in metabolizing the anaphylatoxins; and calmodulin, a calcium binding protein, have all been localized on endothelial cells by immunofluorescence techniques and by functional assays [1, 23, 24, 31]. As shown in figure 1 the localizations are not identical. ATPase (fig. 1 a) and 5′-nucleotidase (fig. 1 b) appear to be restricted to the caveolae, ACE (fig. 1 c) and CPN (fig. 1 d) appear to be present both on undifferentiated portions of the plasma membrane and on caveola membranes. Carbonic anhydrase (fig. 1 e) shows a patchy distribution on the endothelial cell surface. Although not illustrated in figure 1 carbonic anhydrase is also localized in some caveolae and within small vesicles of multivesicular bodies. Calmodulin (fig. 1 f) can be localized in some but not all caveolae.

Thus, caveolae have the effect of increasing the area of cell bound enzymes and are ideally positioned for access to circulating substrates and for return of metabolic products to the circulation. In view of the enzymes that they contain, caveolae, therefore, can be said to play a role in a wide range of physiological functions including blood pressure homeostasis.

Structural Properties of Endothelial Caveolae

Endothelial cells in culture, whether on plastic culture flasks or on microcarriers, are unlikely to be actively involved in the maintenance of barrier functions. Nevertheless, endothelial cells in culture can process bradykinin and angiotensin I to yield the same products as do intact lungs. The cells in culture possess caveolae, and these caveolae contain enzymes, as do endothelial caveolae in situ [15, 19, 29, 31]. Using sensitive assays, we have been able to calculate the number of molecules of ACE and CPN per endothelial cell in culture; these numbers are considerable (bovine pulmonary artery endothelial cells possess approx. 245,000 ACE and 123,000 CPN; while rabbit microvascular endothelial cells possess 205,000 ACE and 4,282,000 CPN [25]). Thus, endothelial cells in culture retain the ability to process vasoactive substances and retain enzymes characteristic of the cell type in vivo. The preservation of these functional

---

Fig. 2. Porcine pulmonary artery endothelial cell in culture showing nucleus (N), perinuclear organelles including Golgi apparatus (G) and mitochondria (M). Caveolae (arrows) are restricted to the periphery of the cell. Bar marker = 1 μm.

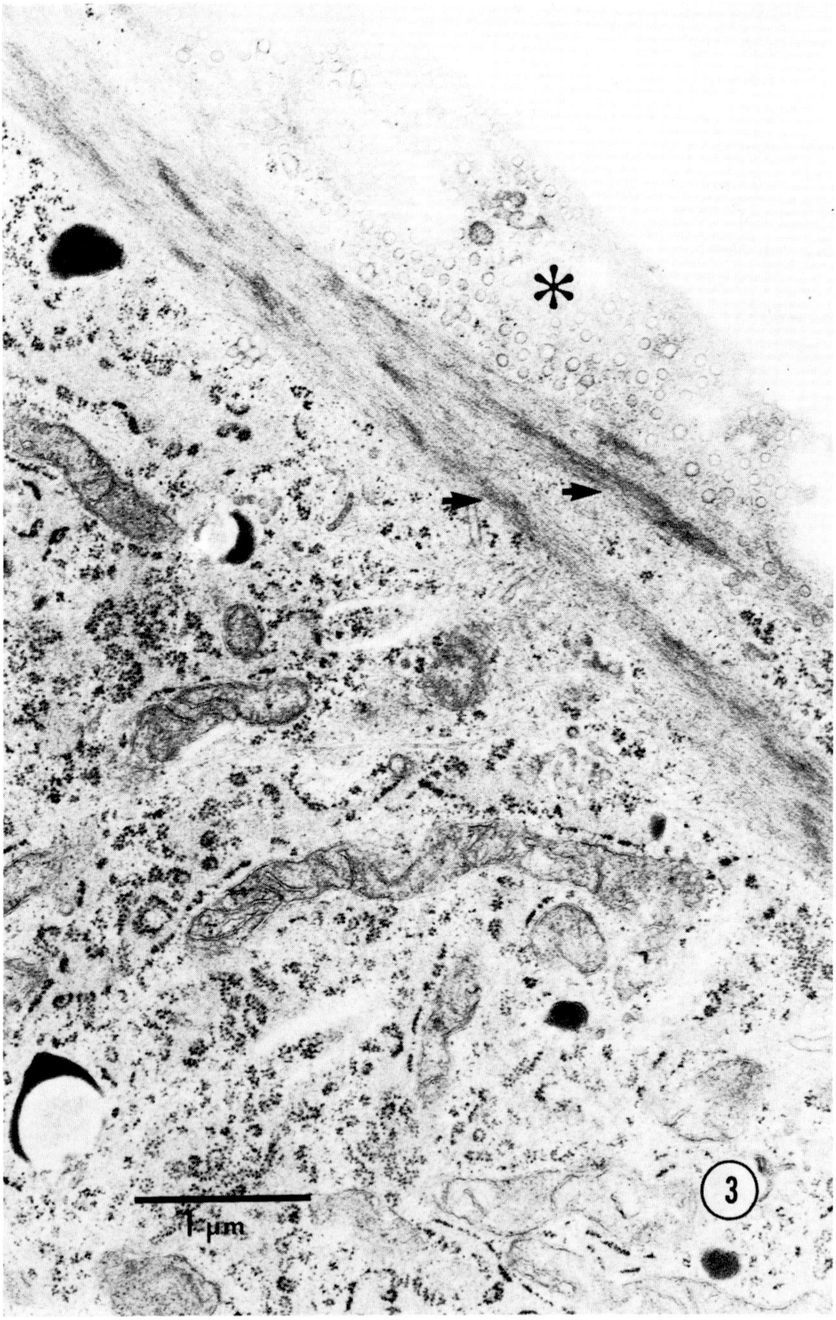
*
3
1 μm

capabilities is matched by the presence of caveolae. When examining caveolae of capillary endothelial cells in situ, the cells are so thin that structures attached to both surfaces, such as caveolae, tend to merge at the center. Endothelial cells in monolayer culture are flat and thin at the edges but are less attenuated than in vivo. In culture, it is clear that the caveolae are restricted to the peripheral portions of the cell. Sometimes (fig. 2), there is simply a layer of caveolae at the periphery while the center of the cell is packed with organelles (including the nucleus). In other instances, the caveolae lie above a zone of microfilaments (fig. 3) that appear to restrict movement. The association of rows of caveolae with microfilaments can be seen by high voltage microscopy of whole unsectioned endothelial cells in culture [27].

One of the advantages of having endothelial cells in culture is that they can be observed while undergoing shape-changes, i.e., during cell division and migration or in response to cell culture techniques for passaging, e.g., rounding up after being removed with a rubber policeman, by EDTA, cold shock or trypsin [6]. When the cells are treated with an injurious substance such as trypsin that removes surface ACE and CPN [23] receptors and junctional proteins [22] and renders the cells more adhesive [2], they round up, and fewer caveolae are found opening to the exterior [6]. Under these circumstances, the caveolae form a labyrinthine system below the surface that may represent a cellular response to protect enzyme sites (fig. 4). As the trypsin is neutralized (i.e., by trypsin inhibitors in serum) the cells resume their flattened shape and eventually resume their enzymatic activities. It is conceivable that the cell can accommodate shape changes (surface to volume ratio changes) by 'banking' caveolae membrane and attached enzymes, that can then be restored to the cell surface rapidly and without requiring new enzyme synthesis and reinsertion of enzyme into the plasma membrane.

Both in culture and in situ caveolae can be found incorporated in endothelial projections, in myoendothelial junctions and occasionally in endothelial – endothelial junctions. These sites suggest that caveolae are a normal component of the endothelial plasma membrane that undergoes the same movement and flow as other components of the plasma mem-

---

Fig. 3. Porcine endothelial cell in culture, similar to that shown in fig. 2, the peripheral zone of caveolae (asterisk) is clearly demarcated by microfibrils (arrows) from the intracellular organelles such as mitochondria and rough endoplasmic reticulum. Bar marker = 1 μm.

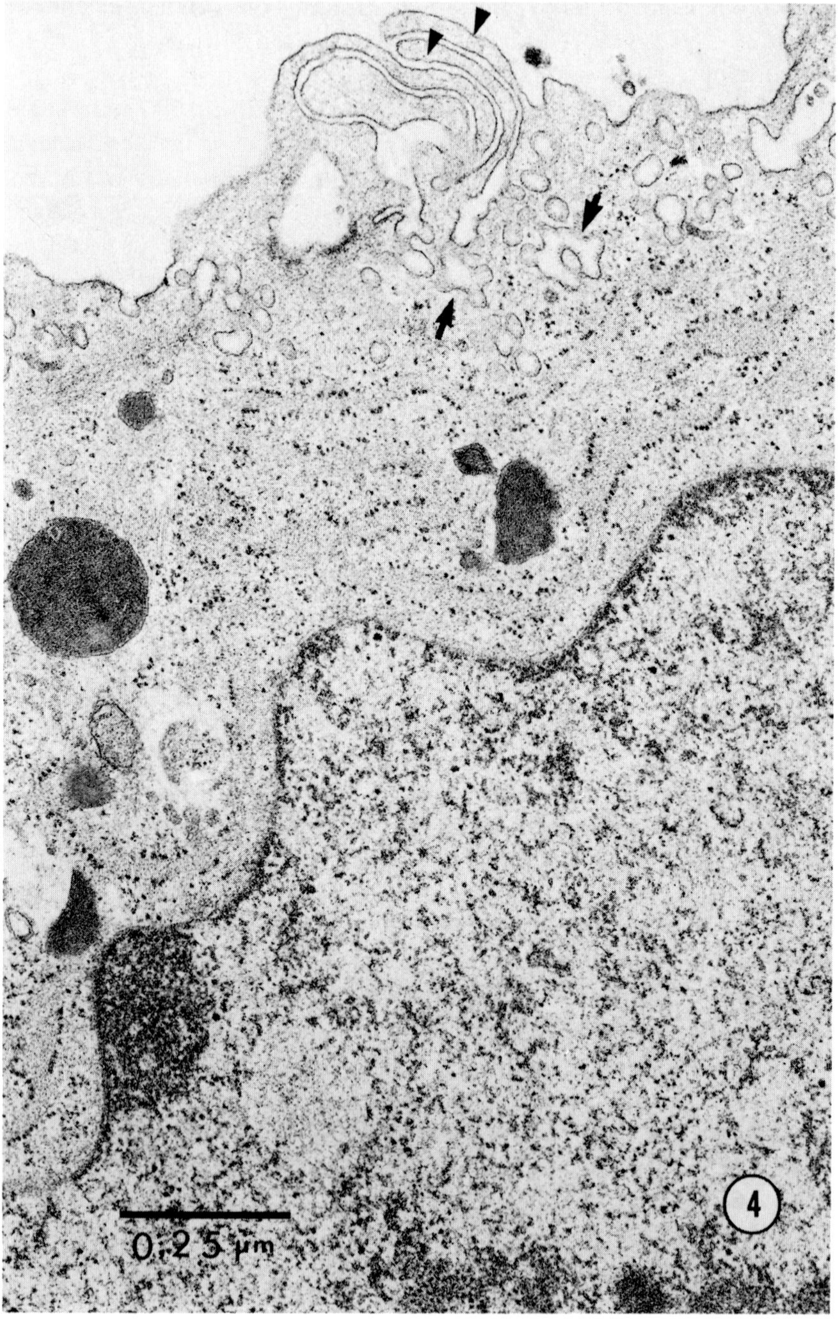
0.25 µm
4

brane. When the plasma membrane is thrown into a projection or forms a junctions, the caveolae too become incorporated in that region.

Both in culture and in situ caveolae are spanned at the luminal stoma by a delicate diaphragm composed of a single lamella [34]. When the caveolae form groups or clusters, diaphragms separate the component caveolae and may be important in maintaining the characteristic shape of the caveolae [34]; the caveolae retain their shape even after plasma membrane fractionation [14, 34].

The diaphragm may be important in providing a microenvironment for interaction of plasma substrates with cell bound enzymes.

All in all, there is evidence that endothelial caveolae are present on both surfaces of endothelial cells in culture, as they are in vivo. Immunocytochemical and cytochemical techniques indicate that enzymes can be localized at those sites that have access to substrate (or antibody), but that sites that are not labeled owing to perfusion of substrates via the vasculature (abluminal surface) do possess enzymes and can be labeled if the tissue is cut into small blocks and soaked in reactants.

Whether endothelial monolayers are fixed before or after incubation with immunologic reagents, there is no evidence that labeled membrane traverses the endothelial cell. Reaction product is restricted to caveolae confluent with the exterior and with direct access to substrate.

Concluding Remarks

The full range of endothelial functions is not known at present, likewise, all the capabilities of caveolae may not yet be recognized. However, it is clear that caveolae provide a means for amplification of the endothelial cell surface and consequently increase the surface area of endothelial enzymes available for processing circulating substances. In addition, caveolae may provide a specialized microenvironment facilitating the selective processing of blood-borne substrates by endothelial cell-bound enzymes. In response to changes in cell shape and in response to injury,

---

Fig. 4. Porcine pulmonary endothelial cell in culture that had been detached from its substratum by exposure to trypsin/EDTA. The cell was circular in profile and caveolae formed a complex system close to the surface (arrows), frequently at the base of infoldings (arrowheads). Bar marker = 0.25 μm.

the caveolae may provide a means whereby the cell can internalize and bank plasma membrane and integral membrane proteins such as enzymes and receptors.

Summary

Physiological studies have indicated that endothelial cells, especially those of the lungs, play an active role in the processing of blood-borne vasoactive substances, including adenine nucleotides, biogenic amines and polypeptide hormones. Studies using cultures of pure lines of pulmonary endothelial cells confirm the hypothesis that circulating ATP, ADP and AMP are metabolized by enzymes on the luminal surface of endothelial cells. Cytochemical localization at the electron microscope level shows that the enzymes responsible are located in those endothelial caveolae that directly face the vascular lumen. Likewise, pure cultures of endothelial cells metabolize bradykinin and angiotensin I to yield the same products as do intact lungs. Immunocytochemical localization at the electron microscope level indicates that angiotensin converting enzyme (EC 3.4.15.1), the enzyme responsible for both degradation of bradykinin and conversion of angiotensin I to angiotensin II, is located on both caveolae and on undifferentiated portions of the endothelial plasma membrane. The enzyme is located with its active site directly accessible to plasma substrates. Endothelial cells in culture provide a means for studying endothelial properties without the complication of enzymic contributions from other cell types. For example, endothelial cells possess, and probably synthesize, surface enzymes such as ATPase, ADPase, 5′-nucleotidase, angiotensin converting enzyme, carboxypeptidase N, and carbonic anyhydrase; enzyme inhibitors such as α_2-macroglobulin; receptors for bradykinin and other hormones; intracellular enzymes for synthesis of prostaglandins and for the synthesis of extracellular products such as components of the glycocalyx and basement membranes. Endothelial cells of the lungs play an active role in determining the quality of systemic arterial blood. Endothelial vesicles that open directly to the vascular space provide an ultrastructural specialization, ideally suited for favoring interaction between solutes and colloids of plasma with endothelial cell-bound enzymes.

Acknowledgment

Supported by Grants from NIH, HL 21568, HL 22896 and from the Council for Tobacco Research, Inc., USA.

References

1 Becker, C. G.; Harpel, P. C.: α_2-Macroglobulin on human vascular endothelium. J. exp. Med. *144:* 1–9 (1976).

2 Brigham, K. L.; Meyrick, B.; Ryan, U. S.: Trypsin induced aggregation of bovine pulmonary artery endothelial cells cultured on microcarriers. Tissue & Cell *16:* 167–172 (1984).

3 Crutchley, D. J.; Eling, T. E.; Anderson, M. W.: ADPase activity of isolated perfused rat lung. Life Sci. *22:* 1413–1420 (1978).

4 Crutchley, D. J.; Ryan, J. W.; Ryan, U. S.; Fisher, G. H.; Paul, S. M.: Effects of bradykinin and its homologs on the metabolism of arachidonate by endothelial cells. Adv. exp. Med. Biol. *156A:* 527–532 (1983).

5 Crutchley, D. J.; Ryan, J. W.; Ryan, U. S.; Fisher, G. H.: Bradykinin-induced release of prostacyclin and thromboxanes from bovine pulmonary artery endothelial cells. Studies with lower homologs and calcium antagonists. Biochim. biophys. Acta *751:* 99–107 (1983).

6 Frøkjær-Jensen, J.; Ryan, U. S.: Reorganization of the plasmalemmal vesicular system during shape changes of endothelial cells in culture. Int. J. Microcirc. Clin. Exp. *3:* 362 (1984).

7 Green, H. N.; Stoner, H. B.: Biological actions of the adenine nucleotides; (H. K. Lewis, London 1950).

8 Ives, H. E.; Schultz, G. S.; Galardy, R. E.; Jamieson, J. D.: Preparation of functional smooth muscle cells from the rabbit aorta. J. exp. Med. *148:* 1400–1413 (1978).

9 Ryan, J. W.: Assay of peptidase and protease enzymes in vivo. Biochem. Pharmac. *32:* 2127–2137 (1983).

10 Ryan, J. W.; Chung, A.; Martin, L. C.; Ryan, U. S.: New substrates for the radioassay of angiotensin converting enzyme of endothelial cells in culture. Tissue & Cell *10:* 555–562 (1978).

11 Ryan, J. W.; Smith, U.: A rapid, simple method for isolating pinocytotic vesicles and plasma membrane of lung. Biochim. biophys. Acta. *249:* 177–180 (1971).

12 Ryan, J. W.; Smith, U.: Metabolism of adenosine 5′-monophosphate during circulation through the lungs. Trans. Ass. Am. Physns *84:* 297–306 (1971).

13 Ryan, J. W.; Smith, U.: The metabolism of angiotensin I by endothelial cells; in Peeters (ed.), Proteides of the biological fluids, no. 20, pp. 379–384 (Pergamon Press, Oxford 1973)

14 Ryan, J. W.; Smith, U.; Niemeyer, R. S.: Angiotensin I: Metabolism by plasma membranes of lung. Science *176:* 64–66 (1972).

15 Ryan, U. S.: Structural bases for metabolic activity. Annu. Rev. Physiol. *44:* 223–239 (1982).

16 Ryan, U. S.: Culture of pulmonary endothelial cells on microcarriers; in Jaffe (ed.), Biology of the endothelial cell, pp. 34–50 (Nijhoff, Gravenhage 1984).

17 Ryan, U. S.: Isolation and culture of pulmonary endothelial cells; Environmental Health Perspectives *56:* 103–114 (1984).

18 Ryan, U. S.: Angiotensin and other peptides; in Fishman, Fisher (eds.), Handbook of Physiology: The respiratory system I, Chapter 10 (1985).

19 Ryan, U. S.; Clements, E.; Habliston, D.; Ryan, J. W.: Isolation and culture of pulmonary endothelial cells. Tissue & Cell *10:* 535–554 (1978).

20 Ryan, U. S.; Lehotay, D. C.; Ryan, J. W.: Effects of bradykinin on pulmonary endothelial cells in culture. Adv. exp. Med. Biol. *156B:* 767–774 (1983).

21 Ryan, U. S.; Mortara, M.; Whitaker, C.: Methods for microcarrier culture and bovine pulmonary artery endothelial cells, avoiding the use of enzymes. Tissue & Cell *12:* 619–635 (1980).

22 Ryan, U. S.; Ryan, J. W.: Vital and functional activities of endothelial cells; in Nossel,

Vogel (eds.), Pathobiology of the endothelial cell, pp. 455–469 (Academic Press, New York 1982).
23 Ryan, U. S.; Ryan, J. W.: Endothelial cells and inflammation; in Ward (ed.), Clinics in laboratory medicine, No. 3, pp. 577–599 (Saunders, Washington 1983).
24 Ryan, U. S.; Ryan, J. W.: Kinins, endothelial cells and calmodulin. Adv. exp. Med. Biol. *156A:* 671–679 (1983).
25 Ryan, U. S.; Ryan, J. W.: Surface properties of pulmonary endothelial cells; in Copley, Seaman (eds.), Surface phenomena in hemorheology; their theoretical, experimental and clinical aspects. Ann. N.Y. Acad. Sci. *416:* 441–456 (1983).
26 Ryan, U. S.; Ryan, J. W.: Isolation and culture of endothelial cells; in Crone, Basset, Sterkers (eds.), New Methods in the study of microcirculation, pp. 1–18 (Paris, INSERM 1983).
27 Ryan, U. S.; Ryan, J. W.: The endothelial cell surface. Biorheology *21:* 39–56 (1984).
28 Ryan, U. S.; Ryan, J. W.: Inflammatory mediators, contraction and endothelial cells; in Courtice, Garlick, Perry (eds.), Progress in Microcirculation Research II (Sydney: Committee in Postgraduate Medical Education, University of New South Wales 1984).
29 Ryan, U. S.; Ryan, J. W.; Whitaker, C.; Chiu, A.: Localization of angiotensin converting enzyme (kininase II). II. Immunocytochemistry and immunofluorescence. Tissue & Cell *8:* 125–146 (1976).
30 Ryan, U. S.; White, L.; Lopez, M.; Ryan, J. W.: Use of microcarriers to isolate and culture pulmonary microvascular endothelium. Tissue & Cell *14:* 597–606 (1982).
31 Ryan, U. S.; Whitney, P. L.; Ryan, J. W.: Localization of carbonic anhydrase on pulmonary endothelial cells. J. appl. Physiol. *53:* 914–919 (1982).
32 Smith, U.; Ryan, J. W.: An electron microscope study of the vascular endothelium as a site for bradykinin and adenosine-5′-triphosphate inactivation in rat lung; in Back, Sicuteri, Rocha de Silva (eds.), Advances in Experimental Medical Biology, No. 8, pp. 249–261 (Plenum Press, New York 1970).
33 Smith, U.; Ryan, J. W.: Pinocytotic vesicles of the pulmonary endothelial cell. Chest *59:* 12S–15S (1971).
34 Smith, U.; Ryan, J. W.: Substructural features of pulmonary endothelial caveolae. Tissue & Cell *4:* 49–54 (1972).

Una S. Ryan, PhD, Department of Medicine D-58, University of Miami, School of Medicine, P.O. Box 016960, Miami, Florida, FL 33101 (USA)

Prog. appl. Microcirc., vol. 9, pp. 165–169 (Karger, Basel 1985)

Discussion of the Presentations: *Pietra, U. Ryan*

WAGNER: One thing that has always bothered me with cytochemical studies, is that after a reaction is done and the preparation is washed, whether or not these caveolae are trapping reaction products, which otherwise might have diffused away.

U. RYAN: I don't think I understand the question.

WAGNER: When you do a cytochemical reaction you get reaction products. The preparation must be washed thereafter. How do we know that the caveolae are not capturing precipitated lead, which otherwise might not been localized anywhere, simply because the vesicles are constrained spaces?

U. RYAN: It's quite possible, but you have to remember the variation in the localization of the enzymes. Some are not restricted to the caveolae and with the same amount of washing you find enzymes on the undifferentiated portions of the cell membrane. In addition, I'm not only presenting visual data, but we have now an enormous amount of assay data on these things, because we can actually count molecules on the cell surface.

WAGNER: But the point you're trying to make in terms of vesicular function is enzyme localization in the caveolae. I have no doubt that there are surface enzymes on these cells.

The second comment refers to the fact that endothelial cells in lung are extremely thin, tenuous membranes. As you already stated there is no room in that cytoplasm for anything more than a few caveolae. Where is the metabolic machinery, e.g., the rough endoplasmic reticulum that is necessary for protein synthesis?

J. RYAN: All this can be found close to the nucleus and there is a large amount of all kind of organelles.

WAGNER: However, there is no comparison to synthetic cells as of, e.g., excretory glands.

U. RYAN: Oh yes, there is, and employing radioactive amino acids you find that these cells produce, e.g., angiotensin converting enzyme, carboxypeptidase N, and fibronectin. The only difference to secretory cells is that EC don't put their products into secretory granules which one can see. But nevertheless they are a true factory.

WAGNER: I'm directing my question primarily to endothelial vesiculae. I have no doubt that once these cells are put in culture they become metabolic factories simply because they need to reproduce themselves.

BASSINGTHWAIGHTE: Dr. *Sparks* and I have been doing some experiments from which we concluded that adenosine is transported more rapidly on the abluminal surface than on the luminal surface of the cell. You have been looking at the 5′-nucleotidase, which presumably is not the translocator, but have you observed any sidedness related to the adenosine?

U. RYAN: Yes. If you do the cytochemistry in intact lungs, the label is restricted to the luminal surface. If you take a block of lung and chop it up so that the reactants have an equal chance of reaching all sides, then you can find the enzyme also on the abluminal surface of the endothelial cell.

SILBERBERG: Do you think that angiotensin and bradykinin are the physiological substrates for those enzymes? And if so, what would they be controlling?

U. RYAN: Yes to the first part of the question. These substances are the naturally occurring substrates for these enzymes that control, among other things, blood pressure.

J. RYAN: There are now about twenty million patients being treated with angiotensin converting enzyme inhibitors and one can really help these people by inhibiting this enzyme indicating that it does control blood pressure!

WILLIAMS: I want to get back to endothelial cells in culture, because that is something that's going to become very important in the next few years. The only true microvascular endothelial cell in culture is one that looks like a microvascular endothelial cell in situ. This slide demonstrates a capillary EC culture from human fat pad which shows these characteristics in that it displays endothelial tubes. This culture, however, differs from other cultures such as yours that it is a nongrowing culture. In addition, these cultures are maintained on basement membrane collagen and yours are on, I guess, plastic. The comment I have may clarify some of the things going on here. An endothelial cell that is growing is a damaged cell and is undergoing inflammatory reactions. Our cells are not growing in culture and they have, therefore, a different metabolism. Similar results may come up in the literature in the next few years, depending on what substrate we culture the endothelial cells. Do you have any ideas to what your cells specifically relate to, capillaries vs. arterial endothelial cells, or how specific can you get with your data?

U. RYAN: I agree that these were derived from capillaries, but they are not cultures. Are they actually not growing?

WILLIAMS: Definitely not, because they are stuck onto the basement membrane, but we can get them to grow again.

U. RYAN: I further agree that what culturists do is very unnatural. They estimate the quality of their culture by how fast the cells divide and I agree that that is a very unnatural situation. However, what we are talking about is microvascular endothelium, i.e., from small vessels, but not only from capillaries. Since we dissect these vessels out we know exactly their size and depending from which side we approach these it is either pre- or postcapillary vessels. They are, in my opinion, not damaged, because one can damage them thereby eliciting FC receptors, the entire inflammatory process and the complement and coagulation systems. If you examine the properties of these ECs over years, the only thing that's abnormal about them is that they are probably dividing more than they would in vivo.

WILLIAMS: My definition, however, of damage is that these cells are growing, and I don't mean that negatively. But an endothelial cell that is growing either, e.g., in inflammation or in wound healing, is not a normal cell, because the mitotic index of endothelial cells is the lowest of any cell in the body.

U. RYAN: I would suggest that our cells are a lot less damaged than yours that have been freshly isolated from a fat pad.

WILLIAMS: But we believe that they are intermediate, because their vesicular transport properties are totally different from the native vs. those grown on type IV or V collagen.

NEES: Cultured endothelial cells are not always growing. When they reach confluence, then they stop DNA synthesis and their autoradiographic index is pretty much comparable to that of ECs in situ.

U. RYAN: We can also arrest growth by changing the constituents of the medium and hold the cells in the incubator for months. I agree that if you make the cells confluent you can also hold them, and you can by simply adding serum induce their growth.

B. Tripathi: Dr. Ryan, have you perfused your endothelial cell cultures constantly and seen a change in your vesicle population or any change in their characteristics?

U. Ryan: The cells that are on microcarriers are being constantly tumbled, which gives a form of flow.

B. Tripathi: Has that changed the caveolae population or any of their properties?

U. Ryan: No. They make a little bit more fibronectin, but otherwise doesn't change their enzyme properties that I've been talking of.

Williams: Referring to cationized ferritin, as a marker, Dr. Pietra, you're using a pI of 9.4–9.5 and if I'm correct the *Simionescus* use a pI of around 8.3–8.4. Is there any difference depending upon the pI of cationized ferritin that's being used?

Pietra: The *Simionescus* used a commercial preparation, which is a mixture of pIs going from 7 to 10.5. We use a preparation from native ferritin with a pI of 7.5, because Dr. *Farquhar* showed in kidneys that 7.6 was highly specific for heparin sulphate. Yet, there is no difference in binding to the vesicles. I have not done quantitative studies, with more or less binding according to the pI.

Clough: We have a range of pIs to up to over 10, and you do see a difference. There seems to be a range of binding and activity sites at the cell surface. The higher the pI the more closely and the more densely ferritin binds to the surface. At the lower pIs, i.e., slightly cationized ferritin you get results similar to those of the *Simionescus*, where you have specific binding sites. If you take the pI higher than you seem to get a uniform layer.

Williams: Some of the differences we have seen may be pI dependent.

Clough: I'm sure they are.

Pietra: I'm not sure they are, because we used a pI of 7.6 and got labelling of vesicles under the same conditions.

Baldwin: I did some work on the rabbit aorta with cationized ferritin in Dr. *Chien*'s laboratory using high pI, about 10. I found that the vesicle diaphragms had a greater affinity for this ferritin than the rest of the membrane. When I reduced the concentration down to 0.01 mg/ml the difference in particle density on the diaphragms compared to elsewhere increased. So there definitely does seem to be a high affinity for this kind of ferritin. I also looked at anionized ferritin (pI of 4.5) and found that vesicle diaphragms had a higher affinity for that too.

PIETRA: This is interesting, because ferritin, which has a pI of 4.5–5, doesn't bind at least in my experience and others. One sees it within the lumen of the vesicles, but I never saw it binding.

BALDWIN: I saw binding, but was using a high concentration of 10 %.

HAMMERSEN: Ladies and Gentlemen, it's written in the program: Concluding Remarks. I don't want to abuse your patience, but please let me make a few statements that came up during this workshop.

I think 'shuttle of vesicles' through the endothelial cells is out forever and we shouldn't take it up again. Another thing that has been shown by many groups here is, that vesicles fuse with each other and that they are connected to both endothelial cell membranes, luminal and abluminal. The dimensions of such vesicular clusters might, however, differ depending upon organ or even species specificities. This is a second reality that we can agree upon.

A possible solution of the problem whether these vesicular clusters might serve as a mechanism for at least macromolecular transport might be as follows: If a single vesicle becomes wedged in between these abluminal and luminal groups of vesicles thereby cross-connecting them for only a fraction of a second, then the data obtained by Drs. CLOUGH and MICHEL would fit with those of Dr. FRØKJÆR-JENSEN. The difficulty, however, resides in the problem, how to identify this 'missing link' that might exist for only an extremely short period of time. To find a solution is up to the physiologists who are so skilled today in developing more and more sophisticated methods and techniques.

I'm obliged to all the speakers for their kind cooperation and I do thank all the discussants who contributed to this workshop which I herewith declare

CLOSED.

Subject Index